A Guide to Oncology
for Veterinary Clinicians
How to Deal with Cancer Patients

Copyright © 2018 Grupo Asís Biomedia, S.L.
Plaza Antonio Beltrán Martínez nº 1, planta 8 - letra I
(Centro empresarial El Trovador)
50002 Zaragoza - Spain

First printing: June 2018

This book has been published originally in Spanish under the title:
Manual de oncología para veterinarios clínicos. Cómo enfrentarse al paciente oncológico
© 2017 Grupo Asís Biomedia, S.L.
ISBN Spanish edition: 978-84-16818-53-2

Translation:
Anne Murray

ISBN: 978-84-17225-42-1
D.L.: Z 1024-2018

Design, layout and printing:
Servet editorial - Grupo Asís Biomedia, S.L.
www.grupoasis.com
info@grupoasis.com

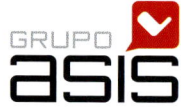

Servet is the publishing house of Grupo Asís

All rights reserved.

Any form of reproduction, distribution, publication or transformation of this book is only permitted with the authorisation of its copyright holders, apart from the exceptions allowed by law. Contact CEDRO (Spanish Centre of Reproduction Rights, www.cedro.org) if you need to photocopy or scan any part of this book (www.conlicencia.com; 0034 91 702 19 70/0034 93 272 04 47).

Warning:

Veterinary science is constantly evolving, as are pharmacology and the other sciences. Inevitably, it is therefore the responsibility of the veterinary surgeon to determine and verify the dosage, the method of administration, the duration of treatment and any possible contraindications to the treatments given to each individual patient, based on his or her professional experience. Neither the publisher nor the author can be held liable for any damage or harm caused to people, animals or properties resulting from the correct or incorrect application of the information contained in this book.

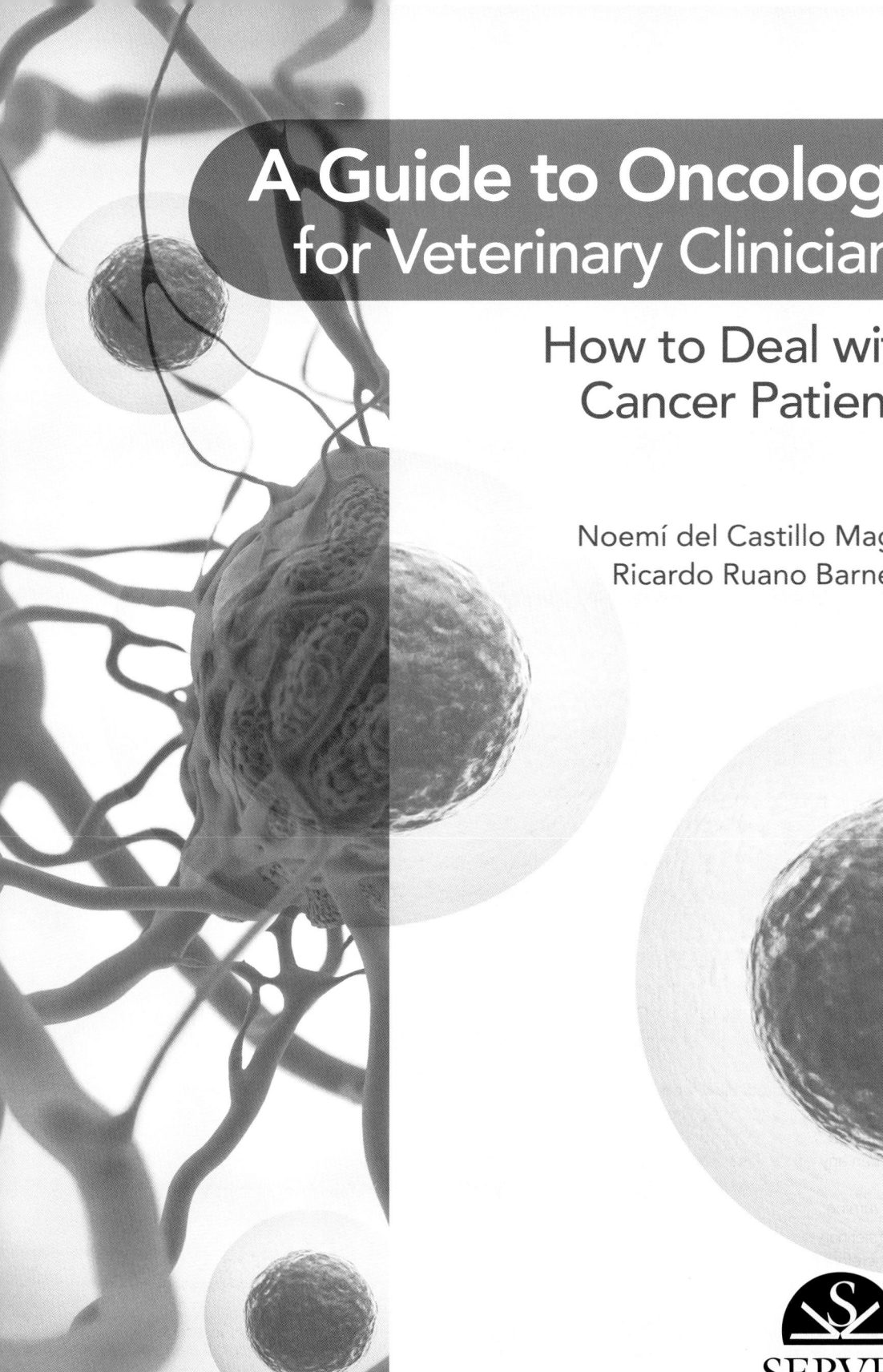

A Guide to Oncology for Veterinary Clinicians

How to Deal with Cancer Patients

Noemí del Castillo Magán
Ricardo Ruano Barneda

SERVET

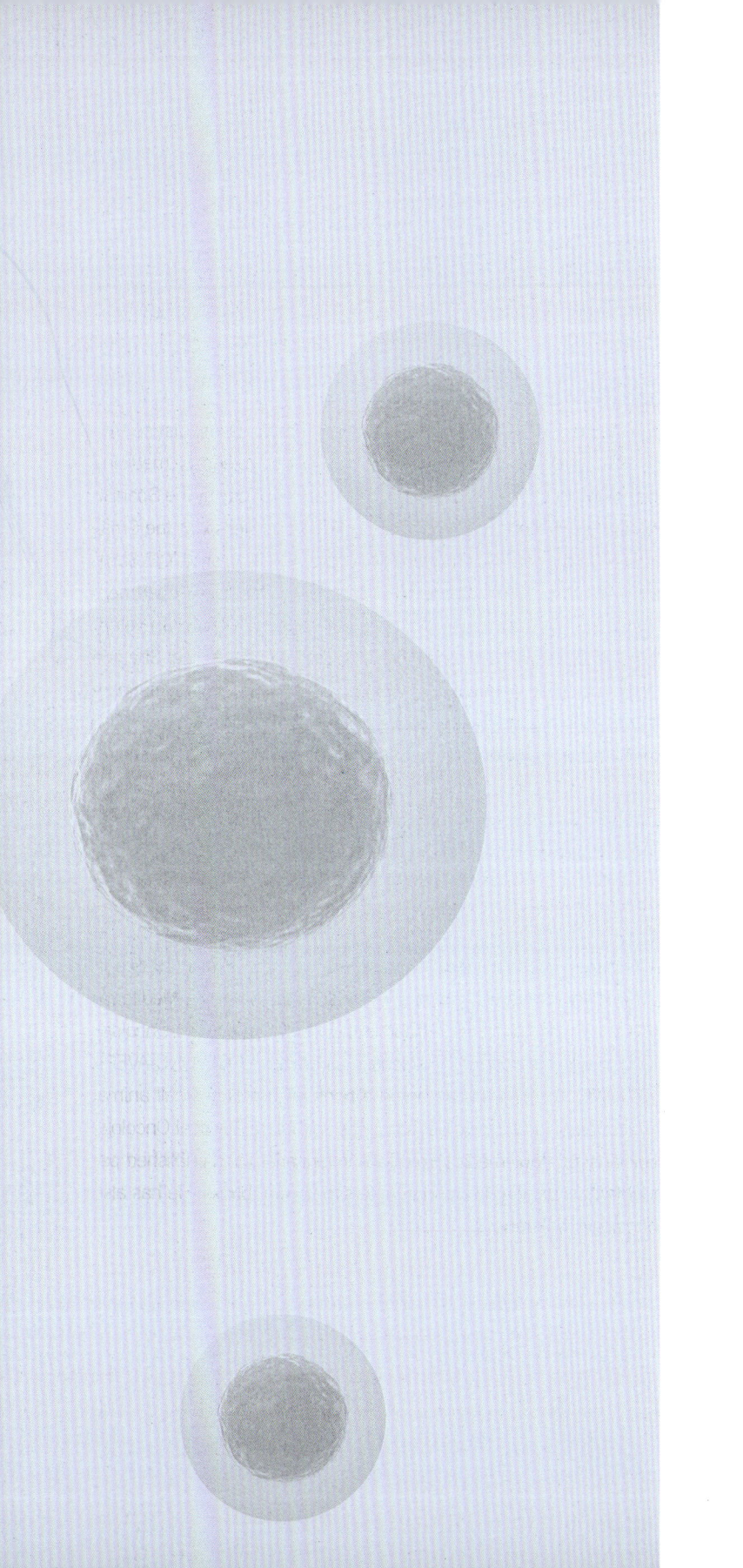

AUTHORS

Noemí del Castillo Magán

Noemí del Castillo Magán graduated in veterinary medicine from the Complutense University of Madrid (UCM), Spain, in 1997 and earned a PhD in veterinary medicine from the same university in 2002. She is certified in veterinary oncology by the Spanish Small Animal Veterinary Association (AVEPA). She has been a professor at the Small Animal Internal Medicine and Anatomical Pathology Department at Alfonso X El Sabio University (UAX) in Madrid since 2005. She is also head of the Oncology Department at the UAX Veterinary Teaching Hospital. In 2004, Noemí joined the Surbatán veterinary clinic as partner and she now heads the Oncology Unit at this practice. She is a founding member of the scientific committee of GEVONC-AVEPA (Group of Veterinary Oncology Specialists of AVEPA), a member of the European Society of Veterinary Oncology (ESVONC), and an honorary member of the Latin American Society of Veterinary Oncology (SLOVET). She has authored and coauthored numerous articles in national and international journals, published chapters in several books, and presented papers at oncology conferences in Spain and abroad.

Ricardo Ruano Barneda

Ricardo Ruano Barneda graduated in veterinary medicine from the UCM in 1999 and is an AVEPA-certified oncology specialist. He is a veterinary surgeon at the Mediterráneo veterinary hospital in Madrid, where he is head of the laboratory and the Oncology Department. He is a founding member of the scientific committee of GEVONC-AVEPA and a member of ESVONC. Ricardo has authored a book on practical small animal oncology *Oncología práctica para el clínico de pequeños animales* (Practical Oncology for Small Animal Clinicians; ed. Multimédica Ediciones Veterinarias) and published papers in Spanish and international journals and chapters in several books. He has also presented work at oncology conferences.

COLLABORATORS

Elena Martínez de Merlo
Elena Martínez de Merlo graduated in veterinary medicine from the UCM in 1987 and earned a PhD in veterinary medicine from the same university in 1993. She has worked as a professor at the UCM's Department of Medicine and Animal Surgery since 1998. She is a veterinary surgeon at the UCM Veterinary Teaching Hospital (HCVC), where she heads the Oncology and Cytology Diagnosis Units within the Clinical Biopathology Department. She has published two books: *Atlas de citología clínica del perro y del gato* (An Atlas of Clinical Cytology in Dogs and Cats) (ed. Servet, 2008) and *Manual práctico de oncología en pequeños animales* (A Practical Small Animal Oncology Manual) (ed. Axón Comunicación, 2011 and 2014). Elena is director of the Continuous Education Diploma in Cytological Interpretation in Small Animals at the UCM, a course which is now in its 10th edition. She is an AVEPA-certified oncology specialist and a member of GEVONC, of which she is a former president. She has presented conference papers both in Spain and internationally and given numerous courses, talks, and practical workshops on oncology and cytological diagnosis. Finally, Elena has authored and coauthored articles on oncology and the application of cytological diagnosis to clinical settings in Spanish and international journals.

Isabel del Portillo Miguel
Isabel del Portillo Miguel graduated in veterinary medicine from the UAX in 2011, where she also participated in a 1-year internship programme and a 2-year residency programme. She joined the UAX's Oncology Department in 2012. She has been a staff member at the Aúna Especialidades Veterinarias veterinary clinic since December 2016. She holds a master's degree in clinical oncology from the Spanish Association of Applied Veterinary Medicine (AEVA) and is currently completing her doctoral thesis on the use of oncolytic viruses in the treatment of spontaneous tumours in dogs.

Josep Pastor Millán
Josep Pastor Millán graduated in veterinary medicine from the Autonomous University of Barcelona (UAB) in 1989 and obtained a PhD in veterinary medicine from the same university in 1994. He has been a professor at the UAB's Department of Animal Medicine and Surgery since 1991, a job he combines with clinical work at the university's Veterinary Teaching Hospital. He is a Diplomate of the European College of Veterinary Clinical Pathology (ECVCP). His areas of interest are haematology and small animal oncology.

Jorge Azcárate Mengual

Jorge Azcárate Mengual graduated in veterinary medicine from the UCM in 1990. He is head of the Diagnostic Imaging Unit of the Mediterráneo veterinary hospital and teaches practical skills at the UCM Veterinary Teaching Hospital.

Ángel Sainz Rodríguez

Ángel Sainz Rodríguez graduated in veterinary medicine from the UCM in 1991 and earned a PhD in veterinary medicine from the same university in 1996. He is a professor in the Department of Medicine and Animal Surgery at the Faculty of Veterinary Medicine of the UCM. He is AVEPA-certified in internal medicine. Ángel has also furthered his training at different centres, including the Veterinary Teaching Hospital at the University of Illinois in Urbana-Champaign, USA. His areas of interest are gastroenterology and endoscopy in small animals and vector-borne diseases, in particular ehrlichiosis and canine leishmaniasis. He is a staff member at the HCVC's Small Animal Internal Medicine Department (specialising in gastroenterology and endoscopy) and head of the Ehrlichiosis Diagnostic Department at the UCM's Faculty of Veterinary Medicine.

Fernando Rodríguez Franco

Fernando Rodríguez Franco earned a degree in veterinary medicine and a PhD in veterinary medicine from the UCM in 1983 and 1990. He has worked as a professor in medicine and animal surgery since 1991 and is head of the Small Animal Gastroenterology and Endoscopy Service at the HCVC. Fernando has been head of the UCM's Animal Medicine and Surgery Department since 2010. He is AVEPA-certified in small animal internal medicine and has published over 90 journal articles and given numerous presentations at Spanish and international congresses. His current research focuses on digestive oncology in small animals and the diagnosis and medical and dietary treatment of chronic immune-mediated digestive disorders.

Andrés Calvo Ibbitson

Andrés Calvo Ibbitson graduated in veterinary medicine from the UCM in 2000. He was a member of the Histology and Anatomical Pathology Department at the UCM's Faculty of Veterinary Medicine from 2001 to 2006, and is currently head pathologist at Citopath Veterinaria. He lectures in histology and anatomical pathology at the UAX's Faculty of Veterinary Medicine.

Ana Cloquell Miró

Ana Cloquell Miró graduated in veterinary medicine from the UAX in 2008. She completed a 1-year internship programme and a 2-year residency programme at this university, where she was active in the Oncology and Neurology Departments. In 2012, she joined the Neurology Department at the UAX's Veterinary Teaching Hospital. Ana has been a resident at the European College of Veterinary Neurology since February 2016. She also teaches neurology-related classes as part of the UAX's Pathophysiology, Diagnostic Imaging, and Clinical Examination modules.

Víctor Domingo Roa

Víctor Domingo Roa graduated in veterinary medicine from the University of Córdoba, Spain, in 2002 and has worked as a small animal veterinary surgeon at the Recuerda veterinary clinic in Granada since 2003. His areas of interest are internal medicine and oncology. He received certification as an oncology specialist from AVEPA in 2013. In 2005, he joined the Tumour Biomarker Research Group at the University of Córdoba, where he obtained his PhD in veterinary medicine. He is a member of ESVONC and a founding member of the scientific committee of GEVONC-AVEPA. He has been head of the Oncology Department at the Hospital Veterinario Sur in Granada since 2014 and in 2015 he joined the Radiotherapy Department at the Centro Integral de Oncología Veterinaria (Cabra, Córdoba), as a veterinary oncology surgeon.

Ignacio Sández Cordero

Ignacio Sández Cordero graduated in veterinary medicine at the UCM in 2000. He is AVEPA-certified in anaesthesia and analgesia. He is also the founder of Sinergia Veterinaria, a company of mobile veterinary specialists that offers services to over 400 veterinary practices and hospitals, mainly in the Community of Madrid. He has headed the Anaesthesiology Department at Sinergia Veterinaria since its creation. Ignacio is a founding member of the Spanish Society of Veterinary Anaesthesia and Analgesia (SEAAV) and served on its board until June 2012. He is currently a member of the board of directors of veterinary specialties at AVEPA. Ignacio has given anesthaesia courses, practical workshops, and online training since 2005 and published over 20 articles on anesthaesia, analgesia, and reanimation in small species in specialist magazines in Spain (*Consulta, Pequeños Animales, Argos, Centro*, etc.) and in specialist online media with an international scope (veterinaria.org, Portal Veterinario). Finally, he has given talks and presented posters at different editions of the National SEAVV Conference.

FOREWORD

As anyone who has worked in this field for some time well knows, current oncological practice bears little resemblance to what it was 10 or 15 years ago. Indeed, veterinary oncology is probably one of the specialties in which most progress has been made in terms of diagnostic techniques and treatment protocols in recent years. Progress, however, has also been evident in the "ownership factor", which itself has driven fundamental developments in the field. Pets are now treated as full members of the family, and owners spare no efforts in making sure that their companions live as long as possible with the best possible quality of life. Furthermore, we will all have had some experience of caring for pets that have themselves provided support to their owners through complicated personal situations.

Today's general small animal veterinary surgeons need basic oncological knowledge to form a correct differential diagnosis and provide essential information on treatment and prognosis to owners of pets with cancer.

Meeting this need is the objective of this book, *A Guide to Oncology for Veterinary Clinicians. How to Deal with Cancer Patients*, a commendable initiative in which I have had the pleasure of participating. The popularity of the earlier version of this guide in Spanish has demonstrated that a quality publication that describes basic protocols for managing cancer patients not only responds to the needs expressed by the veterinary community but is also likely to be extensively used.

There is little doubt that this new edition will fulfil the most demanding expectations, as it provides essential, updated information on diagnosis and treatment (in a field that is constantly changing) in an elegant yet practical format that features colour illustrations and photographs.

Although several experts have participated in writing this guide, Noemí del Castillo Magán, who took overall charge of the project, must take most credit. Nothing Noemí ever does is mediocre and those of us who know her can attest to her professionalism and drive to promote excellence. Her vast experience in the field of oncology, not to mention her excellent teaching skills, is a guarantee that the reader will find this guide to be instructive, useful, and scientifically grounded – in other words, perfect! I highly recommend adding this guide to your bookshelf and am sure that it will become one of the most prized and frequently consulted books in your practice.

Elena M. Martínez de Merlo
February 2017

PREFACE

Oncología clínica: manual de iniciación (Clinical Oncology: A Basic Guide), published in 2009, emerged to meet a growing demand from clinical veterinary surgeons for guidance on how to handle oncological cases. The original book, which I wrote with the help of my colleagues, was a comprehensive compilation of all the information available at the time designed to present clinical veterinary surgeons with a practical framework for systematically managing oncological cases.

This new and improved edition of the guide, which builds on the excellent reception of the earlier version, is coauthored by myself and Ricardo Ruano Barneda, with contributions yet again from a team of reputable collaborators. In this edition we have incorporated aspects that are less widely described in similar publications, drawing on both our extensive experience and the available scientific evidence.

The main aim of the guide is to aid clinical decision-making when dealing with cancer patients and to provide practical guidance for establishing a diagnosis and prognosis and choosing between essential and recommended diagnostic tests. It also explains when to use relatively novel diagnostic techniques (such as flow cytometry and PARR [PCR for Antigen Receptor Rearrangement]), illustrates how to interpret cytology and biopsy results, and describes the biological behaviour of the main cancers encountered in veterinary oncology.

Its six core chapters cover aspects related to communication with owners, clinical signs of different cancers, diagnostic techniques (including cytology, biopsy, flow cytometry, imaging studies, etc), test interpretation and disease staging, treatment (including surgery, chemotherapy, radiation therapy, tyrosine kinase inhibitors, etc), and pain management. Also included are four appendices that provide additional information on paraneoplastic syndromes, chemotherapy protocols, metronomic therapy, and survival according to tumour type and treatment.

TABLE OF CONTENTS

Abbreviations 1

1 Dealing with a patient with a mass: client communication 3
Noemí del Castillo

Introduction 4

Breaking the news and dealing with the consequences 6
    Dispelling fears and myths 6
    Staff training 9
    Losing a pet 9

Quality of life 10

Compassion fatigue 12

2 Recognising signs consistent with cancer in senior pets 13

Signs of oral cancer 16

Signs of skin cancer 17
    Cats 17
    Dogs 18

Signs of abdominal tumours 20
    Cats 20
    Dogs 20

Other signs of cancer 21

Age-related changes in different body systems 22

Diagnosis and prognosis in veterinary oncology 23

3 Diagnostic procedures in veterinary oncology 27

Cytology 28
Elena M. Martínez de Merlo
    Introduction 28
    Sample collection, slide preparation, and staining ... 29
    Cell interpretation protocol 31

Biopsy 32
Isabel del Portillo y Noemí del Castillo

Blood and bone marrow smears 34
Noemí del Castillo

Flow cytometry and PCR for antigen receptor rearrangements 35
Josep Pastor
    The importance of immunophenotyping in canine lymphoma 35
    Flow cytometry 35
    PCR for antigen receptor rearrangements 39

Diagnostic imaging in veterinary oncology 41
Ricardo Ruano y Jorge Azcárate
    Radiography 42
    Ultrasound 45
    Computed tomography 46
    Magnetic resonance imaging 48

Endoscopy 48
    Gastrointestinal endoscopy 48
    Ángel Sainz y Fernando Rodríguez
        Oesophageal tumours 48
        Gastric tumours 49

Tumours of the small intestine	50
Tumours of the large intestine	50
Airway endoscopy	52

Ángel Sainz

Endoscopy in other locations	53

Noemí del Castillo

General state of senior patients. Laboratory tests 54

Isabel del Portillo y Noemí del Castillo

Clinical staging: TNM staging system 55

Noemí del Castillo

4 Diagnostic interpretation, choice of treatment, and prognosis 57

Cytology 58

Elena M. Martínez de Merlo

Cytological assessment of cell lineage	58
Assessment of cytological criteria for malignancy	59
Cytological characteristics of main tumours	61
Epithelial tumours	61
Mesenchymal tumours	62
Round-cell tumours	62
Melanomas	64

Biopsy 64

Noemí del Castillo y Andrés Calvo

What is tumour grade?	65
Tumour margins	65
Special stains	67

Biological behaviour of tumours according to tissue of origin 68

Noemí del Castillo

Epithelial tumours	68
Mesenchymal tumours	68
Haematopoietic tumours	70
Other origins	71

Biological behaviour of tumours according to location 72

Cutaneous and subcutaneous tumours	72

Ricardo Ruano

Epithelial tumours of the epidermis	74
Epithelial follicular tumours	76
Epithelial tumours arising from the sebaceous glands	76
Apocrine gland tumours	78
Mesenchymal tumours of the skin	79
Round-cell cutaneous tumours	80
Head, neck, and ear tumours	83

Noemí del Castillo

Oral cavity tumours	84
Chest cavity tumours	87

Noemí del Castillo

Parenchymal lung tumours	87
Cardiovascular tumours	88
Mediastinal tumours	88
Tumours of the reproductive system	88

Noemí del Castillo

Prostate tumours	88
Testicular tumours	88
Ovarian and uterine tumours	89
Mammary gland tumours	89
Abdominal cavity tumours	89
Canine haemangiosarcoma	89

Ricardo Ruano

Digestive tumours 97	Chemotherapy 120
Noemí del Castillo	*Noemí del Castillo*
Urinary tract tumours 98	Indications 122
Noemí del Castillo	Resistance 122
Nervous system tumours 99	Handling of cytostatics 123
Ana Cloquell	Classification of anticancer drugs ... 124
Intracranial tumours 102	Antibiotics 125
Spinal cord and peripheral	Antimetabolites 125
nerve tumours 103	Alkylating agents 126
Diagnostic procedure 104	Vinca alkaloids 127
Treatment of nervous system tumours ... 106	Platinum-based agents 127
Skeletal tumours 108	Adverse effects of chemotherapy ... 128
Ricardo Ruano	Other 128
Osteosarcoma 108	Iatrogenic Cushing's disease ... 129
Chondrosarcoma 111	Bone marrow toxicity 129
Bone haemangiosarcoma 111	Organ sensitivity 130
Fibrosarcoma 112	Special considerations 131
Multilobular osteochondrosarcoma ... 112	Radiation therapy 132
Synovial sarcoma 112	*Víctor Domingo*
Histiocytic sarcoma 112	Principles of radiobiology 132
Bone metastases 113	Equipment 133
Haematopoietic tumours 113	Indications 135
Noemí del Castillo	Adverse effects 136

5 Cancer treatment 115

Surgery 116	**Antiangiogenic therapy** 137
Ricardo Ruano	*Noemí del Castillo*
Introduction 116	**Tyrosine kinase inhibitors** 138
Indications 118	*Víctor Domingo*
Sample collection 118	Biology 138
Therapeutic surgery 118	Kinase inhibition 141
Palliative surgery 120	Tyrosine kinase inhibitors in veterinary
Types of surgery according to tumour	medicine 141
location 120	**Immunotherapy** 143
	Noemí del Castillo y Víctor Domingo

Biological response modifiers 144	Appendix II. Treatment protocols 162
Recombinant cytokines 144	*Noemí del Castillo*
Antitumour vaccines 144	Canine lymphoma 162
COX-2 inhibitors 145	Induction therapy 162
Noemí del Castillo	Maintenance therapy 164
	Rescue therapy 164
	Feline lymphoma 165
6 Pain in veterinary oncology 147	Induction therapy 165
Ignacio Sández	Maintenance therapy 166
	Rescue therapy 167
Evaluating pain in a patient with cancer 148	Canine haemangiosarcoma/ Soft tissue sarcoma 167
Signs of pain 149	Initiation therapy 167
Pain treatment 152	Maintenance therapy 168
Why treat and when? 152	Multiple myeloma 168
Classification of analgesics 152	Induction therapy 168
New analgesic techniques 154	Reinduction therapy 168
Analgesic treatment during oncological surgery 155	Canine mast cell tumour 168
	Carcinomas in dogs 169
	Carcinomas and sarcomas in cats ... 169
	Osteosarcoma in dogs 169
7 Appendices 159	**Appendix III. Metronomic therapy** .. 169
Appendix I. Paraneoplastic syndromes 160	**Appendix IV. Survival data for nervous system tumours** 170
Ricardo Ruano	*Ana Cloquell Miró*
Haematological disorders 160	
Red blood cells 160	**8 References** 173
White blood cells 161	
Platelets 161	
Metabolic, digestive, and endocrine-related disorders 161	
Cutaneous disorders 162	
Other 162	

Abbreviations

3DCRT: 3-dimensional conformal radiation therapy.

5-FU: 5-fluorouracil.

AC: AC chemotherapy protocol (doxorubicin and cyclophosphamide).

ADC: adenocarcinoma.

AKT or PKB: serine/threonine-specific kinase.

ALK: anaplastic lymphoma kinase.

ALL: acute lymphoblastic leukaemia.

AXL: AXL receptor tyrosine kinase.

BB: biological benefit.

BRAF: protooncogene that encodes the B-Raf protein (a serine/threonine-specific kinase).

BRM: biological response modifiers.

CCNU: lomustine.

CD antigens: cluster of differentiation antigens (e.g. CD3, CD8).

CLL: chronic lymphocytic leukaemia.

COX-2: cyclooxygenase 2.

COXIB: COX-2 inhibitors.

CPX: cyclophosphamide.

CR: complete remission.

CT: computed tomography.

CVP: chemotherapy protocol (cyclophosphamide, vincristine, prednisone).

DMSO: dimethyl sulphoxide.

DXR: doxorubicin.

EGFR: epidermal growth factor receptor (receptor tyrosine kinase family).

EPC: endothelial progenitor cells.

EPHR: Eph receptor (receptor tyrosine kinase family).

FAC: chemotherapy protocol (5-fluorouracil, doxorubicin, cyclophosphamide).

FeLV: feline leukaemia virus.

FGFR: fibroblast growth factor receptor (receptor tyrosine kinase family).

FIV: feline immunodeficiency virus.

Flt3: receptor tyrosine kinase.

FNAB: fine-needle aspiration biopsy.

FNCS: fine-needle capillary sampling.

FSA: fibrosarcoma.

FSV: feline sarcoma virus.

GIST: gastrointestinal stromal tumour.

Gy: Gray (radiation unit).

H&E: haematoxylin–eosin.

HCC: hepatocellular carcinoma.

HSA: haemangiosarcoma.

IHC: immunohistochemical.

IMRT: intensity-modulated radiation therapy.

ISS: injection-site sarcoma.

ITK: tyrosine kinase inhibitor

LMDS: locally multiply damaged sites.

LP: chemotherapy protocol (lomustine, prednisone).

LSA: lymphoma or lymphosarcoma.

LVP: chemotherapy protocol (lomustine, vinblastine, prednisone).

MCT: mast cell tumour.

MDSC: myeloid-derived suppressor cells.

MHC: major histocompatibility complex.

MHC: major histocompatibility complex.

MM: multiple myeloma.

MRI: magnetic resonance imaging.
MTX: mitoxantrone.
NGFR: nerve growth factor receptor (receptor tyrosine kinase family).
NMDA: N-methyl-D-aspartate.
OSA: osteosarcoma.
PARR: PCR for antigen receptor rearrangements
PD: progressive disease.
PDGFR: platelet-derived growth factor receptors (receptor tyrosine kinase family).
PI3K: phosphatidyl inositol-3-kinase.
PNET: primitive neuroectodermal tumour.
PR: partial remission.
PTHrP: parathyroid hormone-related protein.
RUMM: radial, ulna, medial, and musculocutaneous nerve block.

SCC: squamous cell carcinoma.
SD: stable disease.
STB: soft tissue sarcoma.
TAM: tumour-associated macrophage.
TCC: transitional cell carcinoma.
Tie: angiopoietin receptors (receptor tyrosine kinase family).
TK: tyrosine kinase
TNM: tumour–node–metastasis cancer staging system.
TVT: transmissible venereal tumour.
UPC: urine protein to creatinine ratio.
VAC: chemotherapy protocol (vincristine, doxorubicin, cyclophosphamide).
VEGFR: vascular endothelial growth factor receptor (receptor tyrosine kinase family).
VB: vinblastine
VC: vincristine

1

Dealing with a patient with a mass: client communication

Introduction

Treating senior patients with multiple comorbidities is probably the greatest challenge in veterinary oncology. The incidence of cancer in veterinary medicine is rising, and cancer is now one of the main causes of death in senior patients in Europe, the United States, Australia, and Japan. The relationship between pets and their owners has also changed in recent years, and many pets are now seen as part of the family. More and more cats and dogs are thus being treated for cancer and owners are becoming increasingly demanding when it comes to diagnostic and treatment options. Striking the balance between quality of life and treatment is a growing challenge in routine clinical care and is one of the most delicate aspects facing oncological veterinary surgeons. When assessing quality of life and prognosis in a patient with cancer, it is essential to take into account concomitant age-related conditions, such as heart disease, kidney disease, liver disease, and arthritis (Fig. 1).

Age is a condition, not a disease. Ageing involves a series of changes typically characterised by the accumulation of toxins, a tendency towards obesity, organ failure, loss of immune function, and an increased risk of endocrine-related diseases and arthritis. Contemplation of age and ageing is particularly important in clinical practice, as it guides the development of animal health and well-being programmes and the implementation of preventive strategies (mainly in predisposed breeds).

A diagnosis of cancer generally serves to strengthen the bond between a pet and its owner. The relationship between an owner and the veterinary surgeon must thus be built on trust, as if it is not, the outcome will most likely be unsatisfactory for all parties (Fig. 2).

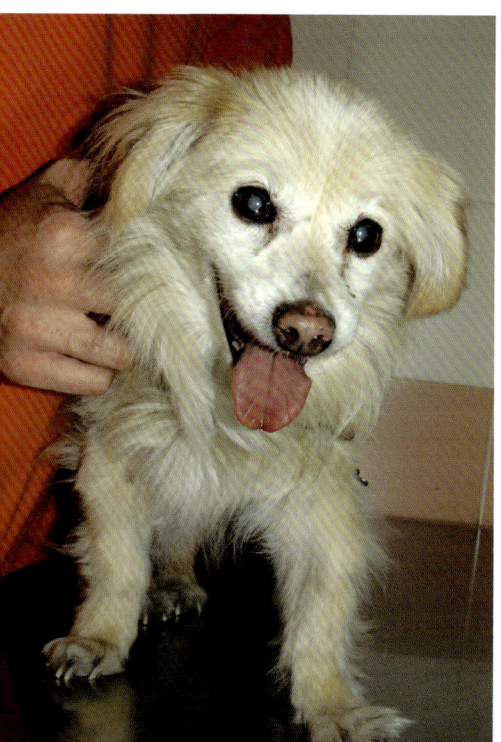

Figure 1. Fourteen-year-old mixed-breed dog with a grade II–III cutaneous mast cell tumour (diagnosed by fine-needle aspiration biopsy). This elderly patient also had heart and joint disease. Concomitant age-related diseases are an important consideration when it comes to choosing a suitable treatment.

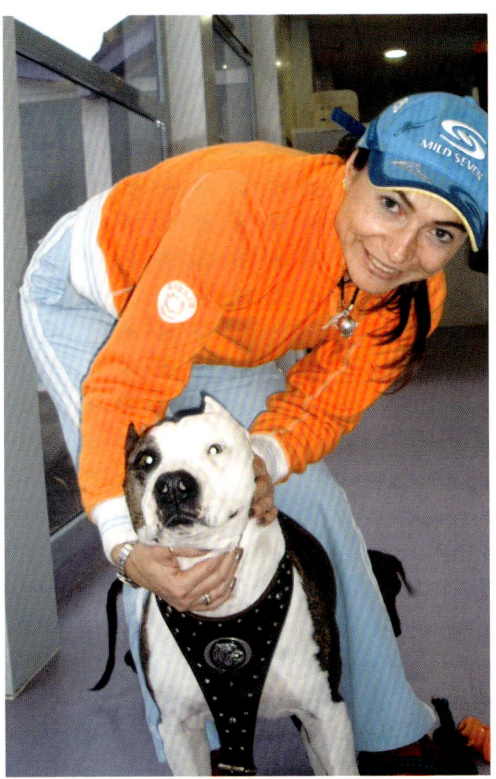 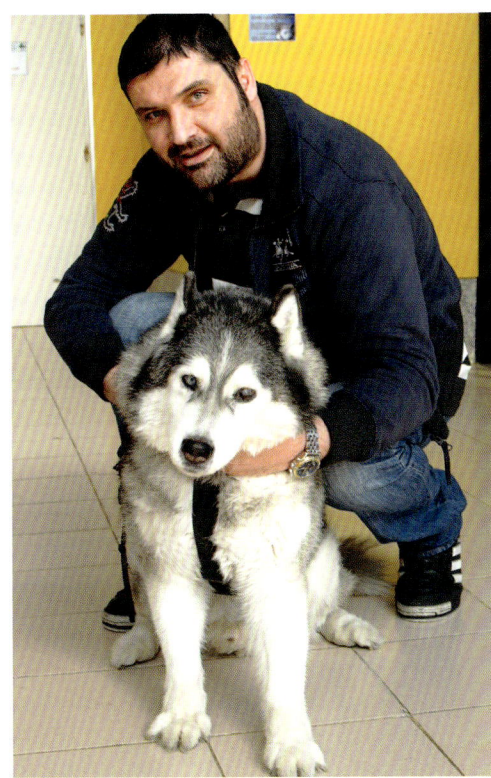

Figure 2. The bond between pets and their owners is often very strong.

One of the main challenges facing any veterinary surgeon dealing with an oncological patient is how and when to treat the cancer. Treatment must be individualised and the veterinary surgeon must be capable of choosing the most suitable diagnostic and therapeutic procedures for each patient, and, from a sociocultural and economic perspective, the patient's family. In the first visit after a cancer diagnosis, the veterinary surgeon is likely to spend most of the time explaining the pet's disease, reassuring the owner, and resolving any doubts. This visit provides the veterinary surgeon with the opportunity to assess the owner's level of involvement, and this information, together with the general condition of the patient, will point to the most suitable treatment.

The greatest difficulty facing veterinary surgeons dealing with oncology patients is probably the existence of preconceptions about cancer and cancer treatment. The words "cancer" and "chemotherapy" are generally scary words that can trigger previous experiences with family members or friends and cause owners to initially reject any treatment due to the fear that their pet will suffer.

Breaking the news and dealing with the consequences

Once the owners have been notified of the diagnosis and given the opportunity to discuss any issues, they must then be given enough time to assimilate the information and take a decision. Unless the patient is in a severe or life-threatening situation, owners should be offered support and sympathy and not forced to take a hasty decision.

This is perhaps one of the most delicate and crucial aspects of dealing with clients, as fear of their companion suffering causes many owners to initially reject treatment. It is important that owners understand that both they and the veterinary surgeon have the same goal, which, apart from curing the animal, is to ensure a good quality of life ("our goal is to ensure that Ron lives a good life for as long as possible").

"The human–animal bond is a mutually beneficial and dynamic relationship between people and animals that is influenced by behaviors that are essential to the health and well-being of both. This includes, but is not limited to, emotional, psychological, and physical interactions of people, animals, and the environment. The veterinarian's role in the human–animal bond is to maximise the potentials of this relationship between people and animals." (AMVA, 1988).

As such, how a diagnosis is relayed to an owner is as important as the diagnosis itself. Veterinary surgeons need to have sufficient tact and psychological insight to ensure that the owner is receptive to the news and the different treatment options available. Again, it is important to reinforce the idea throughout the conversation that the owner and the veterinary surgeon share the same goal, which is to ensure that the patient retains a good quality of life and does not suffer. It is also important to stress the importance of remaining positive, as the patient will improve once treatment is started.

Dispelling fears and myths

One of the goals of any first visit is to analyse the family situation and assess the owner's level of attention. Any doubts should be clarified and the family should be given enough time to analyse the best option for their companion. Consideration must also be given to concomitant conditions typically found in these mostly senior patients when it comes to choosing a treatment and ensuring the main goal, which is a good quality of life.

Engagement of the family in this shared goal is crucial if the treatment is to succeed and if the family is to remember their pet's last months with joy rather than sadness.

Attention should therefore be paid to both verbal and body language when delivering the news, and it is also important to create a climate of trust and make the owner feel part of the team.

Common questions asked by families when they learn that their pet has cancer.
- **Why does my pet have cancer? What have I done wrong?**
  This first question is probably one of the most common questions asked during a first visit, and it is not easy to answer as cancer is normally caused by a combination of genetic and environmental factors. Most cancers are the result of genetic mutations that occur over a patient's lifetime. These somatic mutations can be the result of internal factors (e.g. hormones) or external factors (e.g. exposure to chemicals or ultraviolet radiation).
- **Will my pet get better?**
  The answer to this question will depend on the type of cancer. In the case of treatable but incurable cancers, the objective is to transform the cancer into a chronic disease (like arthritis) by providing treatment that improves both quality of life and life expectancy (Fig. 3).

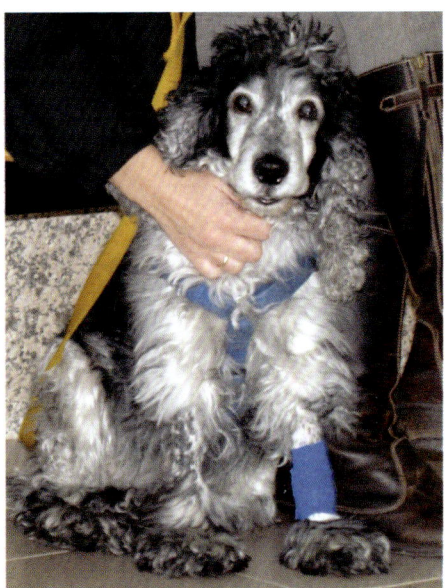

Figure 3. The ultimate goal of many cancer treatments is to transform the cancer into a chronic disease (just like chronic kidney disease, arthritis, heart disease etc.) while maintaining an excellent quality of life and improving prognosis.

- **What will happen if I do nothing?**
  In this case, owners should be informed that their pet will need symptomatic, palliative treatment for as long as it has a good quality of life. Euthanasia should be contemplated once the pet can no longer lead a normal life.
- **Can I use food supplements or alternative therapies while my pet is being treated?**
  The use of food supplements or alternative treatments should be carefully weighed up as these can interact negatively with cancer drugs by altering the enzymes needed to deliver them to their target. Research, however, is still lacking in this area.

There is ample evidence that pet owners go through different emotional states during their pet's illness.
- **Denial.** Many owners initially refuse to accept the diagnosis. In such cases, the veterinary surgeon should be empathetic and convey the necessary information gradually, making sure that the owner is listening and understanding the terms used during the conversation. In some cases it can be useful to give the owners written information on the disease, to put them in contact with other families who have been through a similar situation, or to suggest that they make a list of any questions at home to discuss at the next visit.
- **Euphoria.** Once treatment is started, many owners notice a considerable improvement in their pet, frequently leading them to think that their pet has been given a new lease of life and that the diagnosis was wrong and that their pet is one of these "miraculous exceptions". It is important at this stage to remind the owner that their pet is still unwell, but that the goal of restoring a good quality of life has been achieved.
- **Nonacceptance.** This is a delicate stage, as seeing their pet take a turn for the worse, after apparently being back on the road to recovery, can bring back the negative emotions experienced at the beginning of the process. It is the veterinary surgeon's duty to support the family during this stage and to help them decide when it is time to "let go".
- **Depression.** Losing a pet can leave a large void in families, particularly considering the enormous emotional and physical challenges involved in caring for a pet with cancer. Most owners will appreciate receiving a sympathetic phone call or email, or even a card with the pawprint of their pet during this upsetting time.

Staff training

Pet owners should perceive a general climate of trust and support throughout the veterinary practice. If they receive conflicting information from different members of staff, they will find it more difficult to take a decision and may even choose to take their pet to another practice where they believe the staff work more as a united team.

Losing a pet

The loss of a pet is a difficult moment and the emotions felt at this time can directly influence an owner's overall perception of the care process. Where possible, the decision to stop treatment should be broached with tact and time (Fig. 4). This will help the family to come around to the idea and prepare for saying goodbye and deciding what to do with the remains (individual or mass cremation, burial). Scheduled euthanasias should be planned in a quiet, intimate setting, and owners must be reassured that their pet will not suffer. Once the euthanasia has been performed, the owners should be given sufficient time alone with their pet to say goodbye. Water, tissues, and even a hug will probably be appreciated. It is important to reassure the family at this time and to let them know that it is normal for them to feel sad (they have, after all, lost a member of their family) and that they will all experience the process differently and for different lengths of time.

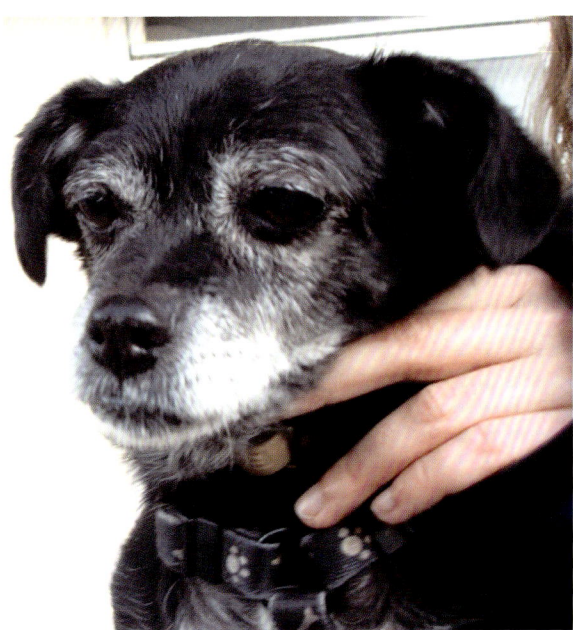

Figure 4. It is very difficult to know when the time has come to end a patient's life. The veterinary surgeon has a central role in guiding this decision and ensuring that the process is as minimally traumatic as possible.

Quality of life

The concept of quality of life has been extensively studied in human medicine, but it is a relatively new concept in veterinary medicine and has probably received little attention to date partly because of the difficulty of evaluating an animal's quality of life. In veterinary oncology, the concept of quality of life is related to the extent to which a patient's organs and well-being are affected by both the cancer and the treatments received. Monitoring quality of life throughout treatment can improve the communication between a patient and the veterinary surgeon, and this in turn can have a direct impact on subsequent decisions regarding a range of aspects such as the choice of treatments to improve quality of life and prognosis (Figs. 5–6).

Score		Criterion
1–10		**Hurt.** Adequate pain control, including breathing ability, is first and foremost on the scale. Is the pet's pain successfully managed? Is oxygen necessary?
1–10		**Hunger.** Is the pet eating enough? Does hand feeding help? Does the patient require a feeding tube?
1–10		**Hydration.** Is the patient dehydrated? For patients not drinking enough, use subcutaneous fluids once or twice daily to supplement fluid intake.
1–10		**Hygiene.** The patient should be kept brushed and cleaned, particularly after elimination. Avoid pressure sores and keep all wounds clean.
1–10		**Happiness.** Does the pet express joy and interest? Is he/she responsive to things around him/her (family, toys, etc)? Is the pet depressed, lonely, anxious, bored, or afraid? Can the pet's bed be close to the family activities and not be isolated?
1–10		**Mobility.** Can the patient get up without assistance? Does the pet need human or mechanical help (e.g. a cart)? Does he/she feel like going for a walk? Is he/she having seizures or stumbling? (Some caregivers feel euthanasia is preferable to amputation, yet an animal who has limited mobility but is still alert and responsive can have a good quality of life as long as his caregivers are committed to helping him/her.)
1–10		**More good days than bad days.** When there are too many bad days in a row, quality of life is too compromised. When a healthy human–animal bond is no longer possible, the caretaker must be made aware the end is near. The decision needs to be made if the pet is suffering. If death comes peacefully and painlessly, that is okay.
Total		* A total of 35 points or greater is acceptable for a good quality of life.

Figure 5. Scale designed by Dr Alice Villalobos to assess patient quality of life and to decide whether a treatment might be successful or whether it should be interrupted. Adapted from *Canine and feline geriatric oncology. Honouring the human–animal bond*. Alice Villalobos and Laurie Kaplan. Blackwell Publishing. 2007

CANCER TREATMENT QUESTIONNAIRE

Survey date _____ Pet owner _____
Name of person completing survey _____
Pet name _____ Weight _____ Species _____

Instructions: Please indicate your assessment by circling the number on the scale next to each question, providing your opinion on your pet's CURRENT status.

Example: 1 2 3 4 (5)

	Disagree		Neutral		Agree
Happiness					
My pet wants to play	1	2	3	4	5
My pet responds to my presence	1	2	3	4	5
My pet enjoys life	1	2	3	4	5
Mental status					
My pet has more good days than bad days	1	2	3	4	5
My pet sleeps more, is awake less	1	2	3	4	5
My pet is dull or depressed, not alert	1	2	3	4	5
Pain					
My pet is in pain	1	2	3	4	5
My pet pants frequently, even at rest	1	2	3	4	5
My pet occasionally shakes or trembles	1	2	3	4	5
Appetite					
My pet eats the usual amount of food	1	2	3	4	5
My pet acts nauseous or vomits	1	2	3	4	5
My pet eats treats/snacks	1	2	3	4	5
Hygiene					
My pet keeps him/herself clean	1	2	3	4	5
My pet smells like urine or has skin irritation	1	2	3	4	5
My pet's hair is greasy, matted, rough looking	1	2	3	4	5
Water intake (hydration)					
My pet drinks adequately	1	2	3	4	5
My pet has diarrhoea	1	2	3	4	5
My pet is urinating a normal amount	1	2	3	4	5
Mobility					
My pet moves normally	1	2	3	4	5
My pet lies in one place all day long	1	2	3	4	5
My pet is as active as he/she has always been	1	2	3	4	5
General health					
General health compared to last assessment	1	2	3	4	5
	Worse		Same		Better
General health compared to initial diagnosis of cancer	1	2	3	4	5
	Worse		Same		Better
Current quality of life	Very poor	—	—	—	Excellent

Figure 6. Cancer treatment survey, designed to evaluate quality of life in cats and dogs with cancer. Adapted from Lynch et al., 2010.

Compassion fatigue

High levels of emotional strain are common across all health care disciplines, and veterinary medicine is no exception.

Compassion fatigue is an unavoidable consequence of empathy and compassion. It is caused by a depletion in the veterinary surgeon's emotional resources over time and is frequently confused with burnout. It cannot be predicted and signs include a loss of interest, less enthusiasm for the profession, and physical and psychological disorders. Burnout, by contrast, is predictable and is related to physical and mental exhaustion rather than emotional exhaustion and a loss of energy. Compassion fatigue can affect veterinary surgeons of any sex or age, but oddly enough it appears to mainly affect people at the height of their careers.

Compassion fatigue is one of the main reasons for quitting the veterinary profession and it is therefore essential to recognise its signs before it becomes a problem.

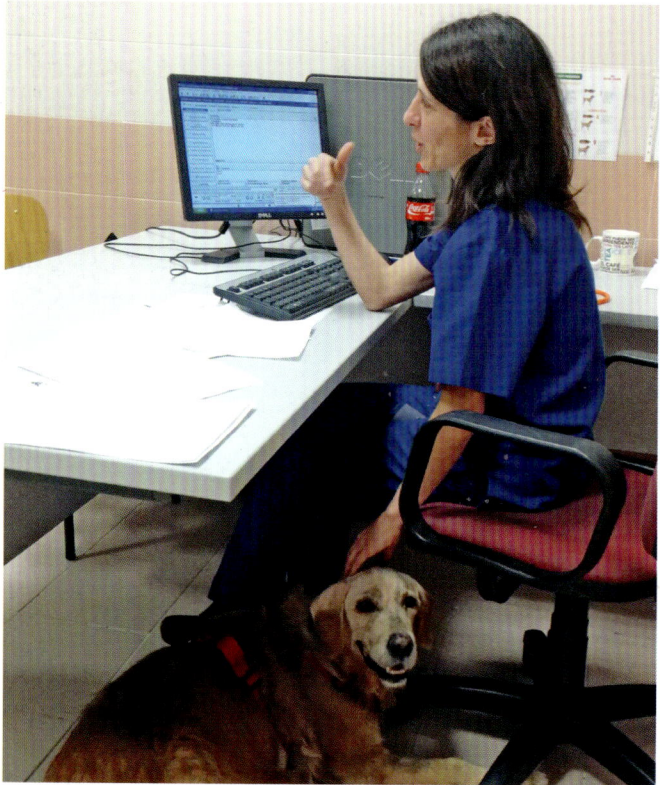

Figure 7. Dealing with pets with terminal disease is one of the factors that may lead to compassion fatigue.

2

Recognising signs consistent with cancer in senior pets

There are cases in which cancer is sometimes relatively easy to recognise or suspect (e.g. a patient with a cutaneous mass). Many signs of cancer, however, can be masked by other conditions, such as obesity, arthrosis, or periodontal disease. In cases with no associated clinical signs, tumours in certain body cavities may go unnoticed, while in others, paraneoplastic syndromes may precede the diagnosis of the primary tumour.

As early detection is directly linked to prognosis, every effort should be made to establish a diagnosis as soon as possible. It is therefore important to perform regular check-ups in geriatric patients and to be familiar with the signs associated with cancer.

These signs can be classified into the following groups (adapted from Villalobos, A., 2007):

- **Palpable signs**
    - Enlarged lymph nodes (Fig. 1), abnormal inflammation, cutaneous plaques with uncontrolled growth.
    - Oral cavity, mammary gland (Fig. 2), testicle, and vaccination-site masses, enlarged organs (abdominal palpation).
    - Wounds or ulcers that fail to heal (particularly in animals with a white coat).
- **Alarming physiological changes**
    - Weight loss, cachexia (Fig. 3).
    - Pale mucous membranes, jaundice, lameness, mucosal hyperaemia.
    - Abdominal swelling, organomegaly, ascites, haemoabdomen.
    - Petechiae (Fig. 4), ecchymosis, spontaneous bleeding.
- **Changes in pet's routine**
    - Anorexia.
    - Loss of energy, lower exercise tolerance, dyspnoea, coughing.
    - Dysphagia, hypersalivation, regurgitation, voice changes, vomiting.
    - Chronic sneezing, chronic eye discharge, unilateral nasal discharge.
    - Dysuria, stranguria, persistent haematuria.
    - Diarrhoea, tenesmus, constipation, haematochezia, changes in faeces.
    - Lameness, joint pain on movement (Fig. 5), hesitation to exercise.
    - Polyuria/polydipsia in the absence of chronic kidney disease, endocrine-related diseases, hypercalcaemia, and liver disease.
    - Syncope, decreased heart sounds, pericardial effusion, pleural effusion, tachypnoea.
    - Weakness, ataxia, paresis, behavioural changes, and pain.

Recognising signs consistent with cancer in senior pets

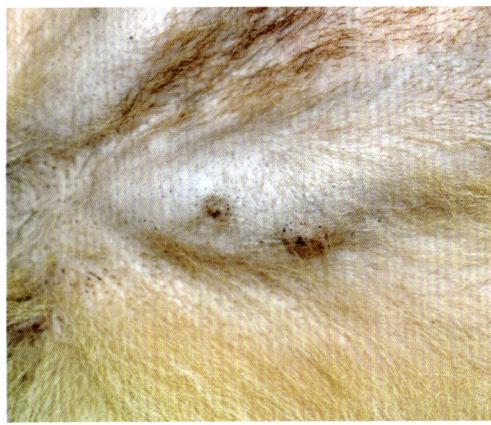

Figure 1. Enlarged inguinal lymph nodes in a dog with multicentric lymphoma.

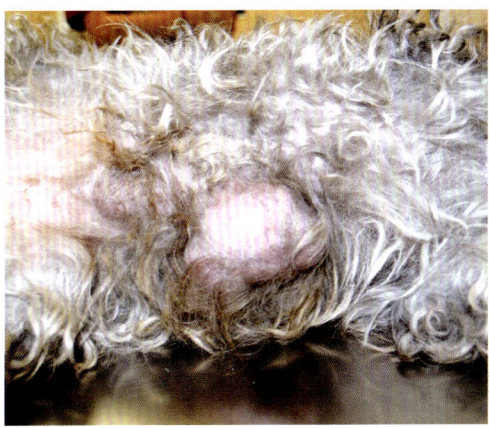

Figure 2. Masses consistent with mammary tumours in a 14-year-old nonspayed female dog.

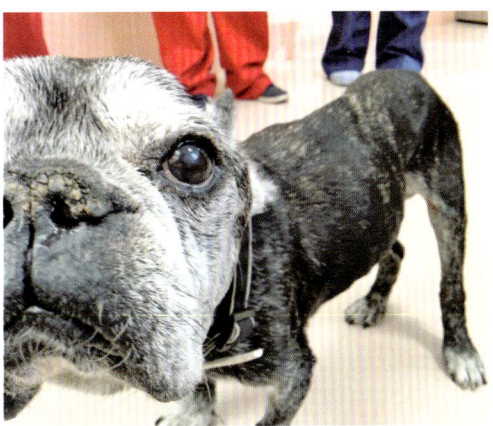

Figure 3. Extreme cachexia.

The presenting signs of cancer are similar to those seen in many degenerative age-related diseases and this can make early diagnosis particularly challenging. Special attention should be paid to remarks by owners about changes in their pet's behaviour, particularly when there are no obvious explanations.

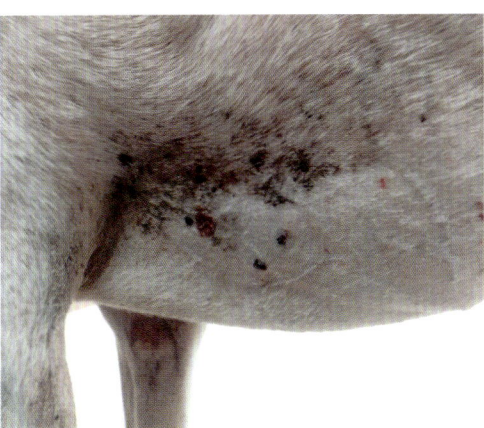

Figure 4. Skin lesions consistent with petechiae histologically diagnosed as cutaneous haemangiosarcoma.

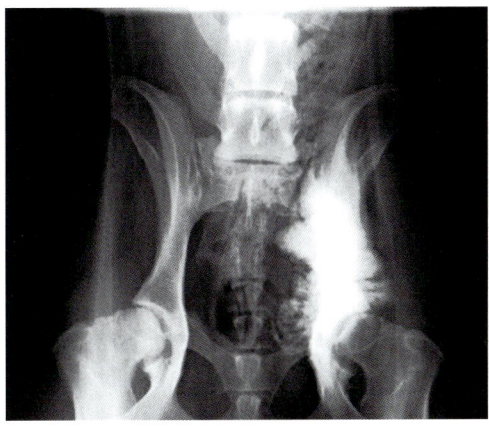

Figure 5. Proliferative lesion consistent with osteosarcoma on the hip of a dog.

Signs of oral cancer

The main signs associated with oral cancer are:
- Hypersalivation, mouth pain, traces of blood in the pet's food or water bowl (Figs. 6 and 7).
- Chewing on one side of the mouth, spitting out of food, difficulty holding objects in the mouth.
- Dysphagia, anomalous movements of the tongue while chewing.
- In the case of cats, failure to eat despite interest in food.
- Halitosis.

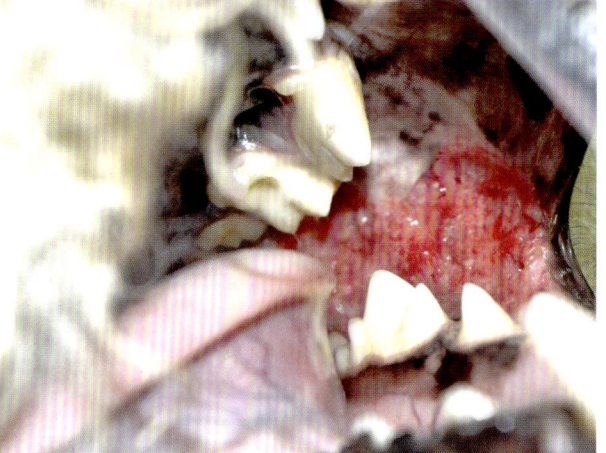

Figure 6. Lesion consistent with squamous cell carcinoma on the palate of a dog.

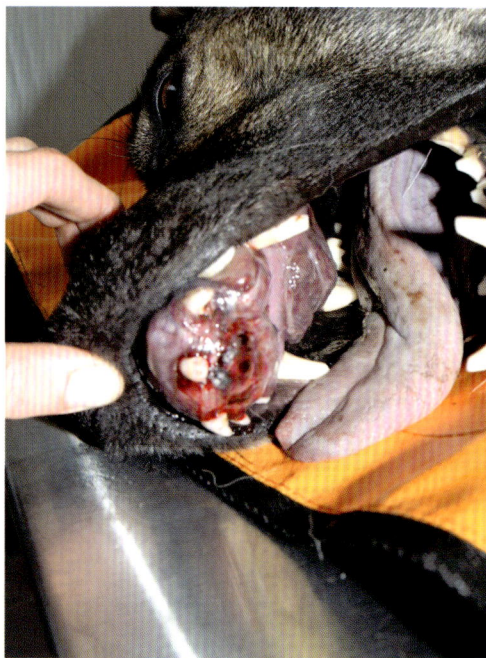

Figure 7. A dog with oral cancer. The patient had anorexia and traces of blood in the saliva (two common signs of oral cancer).

The most common oral cavity tumours are squamous cell carcinoma (SCC), epulis, fibrosarcoma, and chondrosarcoma. The choice of surgical and/or medical treatment will depend mainly on the location and the extent of the tumour (clinical stage).

Signs of skin cancer

Cats

With the exception of feline injection site–sarcoma (ISS), cats are much less likely to develop skin cancer than dogs.

Benign tumours tend to be solitary, well-delimited, nonulcerated lesions that are not adhered to the skin or deeper layers. Surgery is generally curative. Siamese cats appear to have a greater risk of skin cancer.

Most malignant tumours involve the head, shoulder, back, limbs, or mammary glands. They tend to be multiple, poorly delimited, ulcerated, alopecic masses that display invasive growth and are adhered to the skin or deeper layers; there may also be regional lymph node involvement and/or distant metastasis.

When a small nodular lesion is observed at a vaccine injection site (or the injection site of any irritant substance administered subcutaneously [Fig. 8]), the 3-2-1 rule of the Vaccine-Associated Feline Sarcoma Task Force should be applied. According to this rule, biopsy should be performed to rule out the presence of ISS on detection of:

1. A mass that has been present for longer than 3 months after the injection.
2. A mass that is wider than 2 cm in diameter.
3. A mass that increases in size after 1 month.

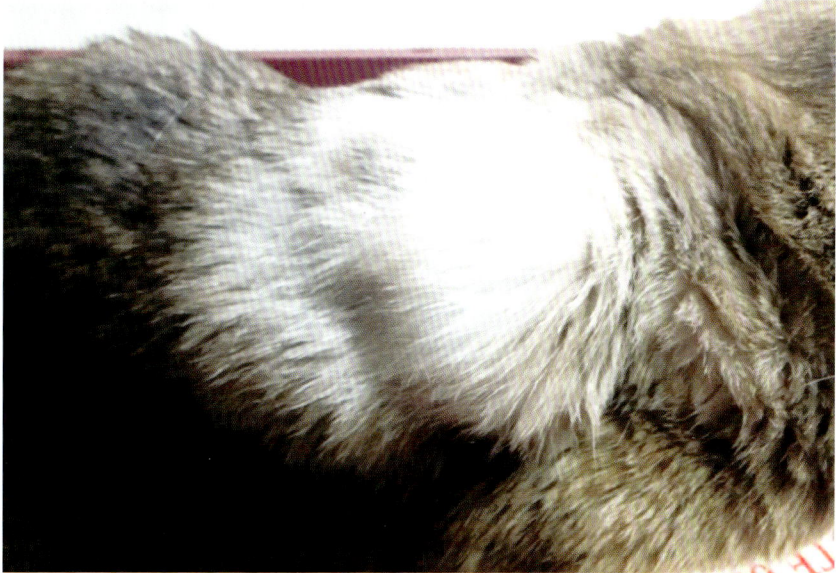

Figure 8. Interscapular mass consistent with feline injection–site sarcoma.

Feline leukaemia virus (FeLV) and feline sarcoma virus are both associated with the development of multiple skin masses in young cats.

Superficial ulcers that do not respond to treatment in poorly pigmented areas in senior cats can indicate the presence of SCC (or carcinoma in situ). The most common locations are the ears, nose, lips, and temporal area.

Dogs

Mast cell tumour. Mast cell tumour is the most common skin tumour in dogs, and it is particularly prevalent in brachycephalic breeds. It can present either as a solitary, well-defined lesion that is not adhered to underlying structures and displays benign behaviour or as an anaplastic tumour with a high potential for spread and a dismal prognosis (Fig. 9).

Squamous cell carcinoma. Dogs with white or lightly pigmented coats that are exposed to high levels of sunlight have a relatively high risk of SCC. This risk may be even greater in Pit Bulls, white Boxers, Dalmatians, and Great Danes with a harlequin coat. Typical presentations include pruritus, chronic inflammation, and ulcers that fail to heal (Fig. 10).

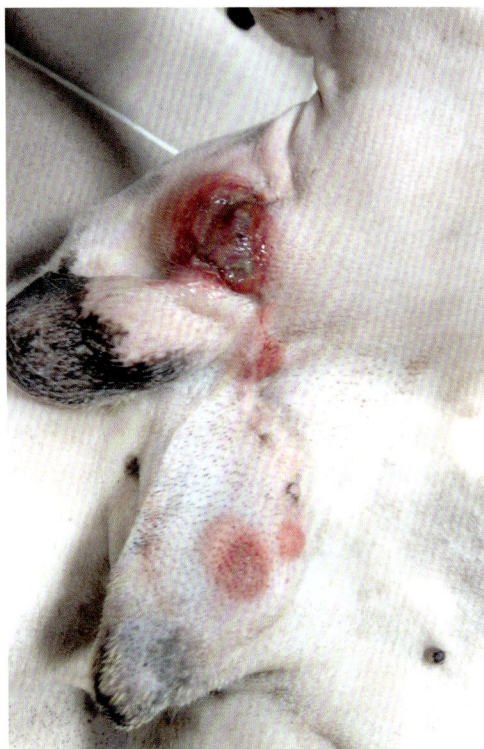

Figure 9. Grade II mast cell tumour in the inguinal area of a male French Bulldog.

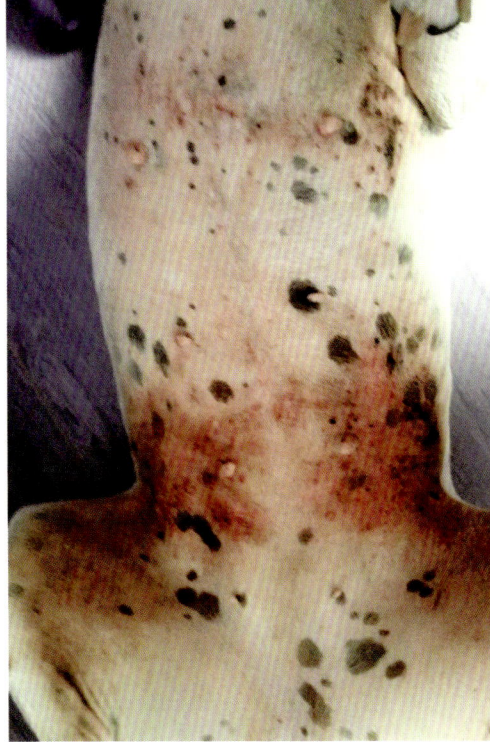

Figure 10. Lesions consistent with SCC on the abdomen of a dog with a white coat.

Haemangiosarcoma. Haemangiosarcoma (HSA) is also common in dogs, and is more prevalent in Pit Bulls, Staffordshire Terriers, Bassett Hounds, Beagles, Dalmatians, white Boxers, and Springer Spaniels. Typical presentations include more or less well-defined single or multiple reddish skin nodules with a soft, cyst-like consistency and flat red patches or collections of blood that are macroscopically difficult to distinguish from a haematoma.

Cutaneous lymphoma. Cutaneous lymphoma or lymphosarcoma (LSA) is the most common form of extranodal lymphosarcoma. It is growing in prevalence and is frequently confused with dermatitis, particularly when it presents as plaques. There are two typical forms of cutaneous lymphoma: nonepitheliotropic lymphoma, which is more common in cats, and epitheliotropic lymphoma or mycosis fungoides (Fig. 11), which is more common in dogs. In the first case, the lesions are located in the dermis or the subcutaneous layers and are similar to solitary or multiple nodules or infiltrative plaques, while in the second case, they are located in the epidermis or adnexal structures.

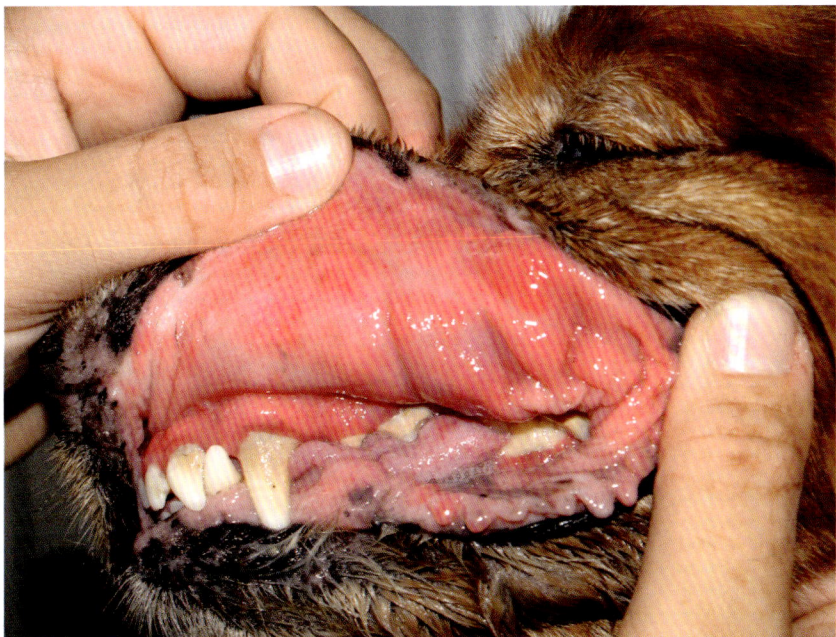

Figure 11. Lesions on the oral mucosa with mucosal thickening in a Cocker Spaniel; the findings were consistent with epitheliotropic cutaneous lymphoma.

Mammary tumours. Mammary tumours are the leading cause of death in non-spayed female dogs. Any nodule observed in the mammary region is potentially malignant and must be investigated.

Signs of abdominal tumours

Abdominal tumours are one of the greatest challenges for veterinary oncologists as they can develop silently. In addition, because they have ample room to spread without causing functional alterations, they are generally diagnosed at an already advanced stage. They may, however, be found during a routine geriatric check-up or during the clinical staging of another disease.

Cats
One of the most common tumours in adult FeLV-negative cats is feline alimentary lymphoma, which can present with highly nonspecific signs ranging from weight loss to alternating diarrhoea and constipation.

Dogs
Splenic tumours are relatively common in dogs. They present with nonspecific clinical signs, and many owners attribute increases in abdominal volume to weight gain resulting from less exercise. Patients are normally brought in for emergency care due to internal bleeding caused by the rupture of a splenic mass. The most common splenic tumour is HSA (Fig. 12), which can also affect the liver and the right atrium. The dogs at highest risk are German Shepherds, crosses with German Shepherds, Golden Retrievers, and medium and large dogs in general.

Primary or metastatic liver tumours can also display similar clinical signs to those observed in splenic masses. Patients tend to have normocytic, normochromic anaemia.

The differential diagnosis in senior patients with haematuria, particularly when this does not respond to treatment, should include urinary tract cancers, such as bladder tumours (transitional cell carcinoma), prostate tumours (prostate carcinoma), and renal parenchymal tumours.

Other abdominal tumours commonly found in dogs are colon tumours, which are accompanied by altered faeces and occasional haematochezia.

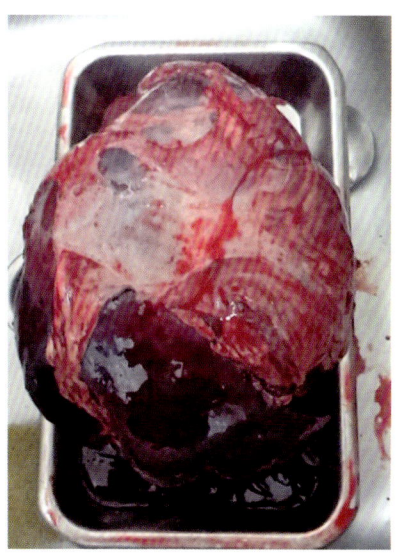

Figure 12. Macroscopic image of a splenic haemangiosarcoma.

Other signs of cancer

Below is a list of other potential signs of cancer, together with their possible cause:
- Acute shock: rupture of an abdominal mass.
- Acute dyspnoea: pleural effusion (particularly in cats with mediastinal lymphosarcoma).
- Pathological fractures: osteosarcoma.
- Acute paresis: spinal cord tumour (primary or metastatic).
- Seizures and behavioural changes: primary or metastatic tumour of the central nervous system.
- Painful mandibular inflammation: oral cavity tumour.
- Weight loss or cachexia without a known cause.
- Paraneoplastic syndromes (see Appendix I). Anaemia within paraneoplastic syndromes. This can be caused by:
  - Chronic disease: normochromic, normocytic.
  - Chronic blood loss: microcytic, hypochromic.
  - Microangiopathy: schistocytes, haemolysis.
  - Immune-mediated diseases: spherocytes, haemolysis, reticulocytes.
  - Myelophthisis (bone marrow invasion): normally associated with leukaemia.
  - Bone marrow hypoplasia: common in Sertoli cell tumours due to hyperestrogenism.
  - Others: hypersplenism, erythrophagocytosis (malignant histiocytosis), or iatrogenic causes (chemotherapy).

Table 1 shows a list of age-related changes potentially suggestive of malignancy organised by body system.

Age-related changes in different body systems

Table 1. Illustration of the multiple age-related conditions that can also indicate the presence of malignancy.

System		
Musculoskeletal system	• Loss of flexibility. • Loss of muscle mass. • Reduced response to stress. • Loss of hair quality. • Foot pad hyperkeratosis. • Fragile nails. • Loss of skin elasticity.	• Collagen granulation and fragmentation. • Hyperplasia of sebaceous and apocrine glands. • Rancid sebum. • Collagen fragmentation and loss of flexibility. • Arthritis, painful joints.
Digestive system	• Periodontal disease. • Reduced salivary secretion. • Reduced oesophageal muscle tone. • Contraction of the cardia. • Reduced secretion of hydrochloric acid, resulting in vomiting, flatulence, and diarrhoea.	• Fatty liver, nodular hyperplasia, cirrhosis. • Reduced secretion of pancreatic enzymes • Reduced absorption of lipids and fats from the gastrointestinal tract (villous atrophy).
Respiratory system	• Chronic bronchitis. • Reduced mucus volume and viscosity. • Ciliary paralysis (less retention of material).	• Increased histamine release (bronchoconstriction). • Respiratory muscle weakness.
Cardiovascular system	• Fibrosis. • Tracheal collapse. • Reduced diffusion of oxygen.	
Kidneys	• Reduced glomerular filtration rate, reduced perfusion, reduced tubular mass. • Thickening of glomerular capillaries. • Ischaemic atrophy and peritumoural fibrosis.	• Hypertension, increased vascular resistance. • Reduced response to antidiuretic hormone. • Reduced erythropoietin secretion. • Shorter erythrocyte half-life due to uraemia.
Urogenital system	• Loss of urethral sphincter tone. • Chronic cystitis, greater risk of urinary tract infections.	
Endocrine system	• Reduced overall hormone secretion. • Reduced sensitivity to thyroid hormone receptors.	• Pendulous prepuce (due to secretion of oestrogens in Sertoli cell tumour). • Androgen deficiency, ovarian involution.
Central nervous system	• Fewer neurotransmitters. • Deafness, blindness, lower tactile sensitivity. • Cognitive dysfunction syndrome. • Behavioural changes.	• Disorientation. • Less social interaction. • Sleep disorders. • Altered or reduced activity.
Immune system	• Lower T-cell density. • Reduced tumour suppressor and repair gene activity.	• Greater risk of neoplasms. • Thymic involution.

Adapted from Alicia Villalobos (2007).

Diagnosis and prognosis in veterinary oncology

When there are firm reasons to suspect cancer, it is essential to follow a systematic procedure to evaluate the pet's quality of life and check for concomitant age-related diseases, such as kidney disease, heart disease, liver disease, and osteoarthritis. If these are not well compensated, they may require treatment.

When examining a dog or cat with a mass or clinical signs associated with cancer, the first step is to distinguish between inflammation and malignancy. If the mass is malignant, the next step is to identify its origin (epithelial, mesenchymal, or round-cell) and growth pattern (localised, infiltrative, slow, fast, etc.), establish an appropriate treatment plan, and determine prognosis by integrating clinical, cytological, and histopathological findings.

A thorough history should be taken during this initial visit to obtain information on the onset and course of disease. The general physical examination should be followed by an oncological examination of the mass (estimation of 3-dimensional volume, connection to other structures, etc.).

Cytology can significantly contribute to establishing a tentative diagnosis during the first visit as it often provides the information needed to differentiate between inflammatory and neoplastic tissue and benign and malignant masses. This simple test also helps to determine the degree of surgical aggressiveness needed and the urgency of treatment.

If the cytology results are inconclusive (the sample may have been taken from necrotic tissue, inflammatory tissue adjacent to the tumour, fat, etc.), extraction of a sample or removal of the mass (via incisional and excisional biopsy, respectively) can help to establish a tentative diagnosis.

TO SUM UP

When faced with a suspected case of cancer, the following steps should be taken:

MEDICAL HISTORY

- Time of tumour onset and appearance at onset.
- Location.
- Growth rate and relationship with other vital structures.
- Pruritus, ulceration, changes in size.
- Previous treatments and responses.
- Presence of paraneoplastic syndromes.

PHYSICAL EXAMINATION

- General health of the animal.
- Identification and characterisation of primary tumour: location, 3-dimensional volume, type of growth (invasive, encapsulated, well/poorly defined), rate of growth (slow, stationary, rapid), relationship with other vital organs/structures, adherence to deeper and superficial layers. This information will give an indication of the biological behaviour of the tumour.
- Regional lymph nodes and possible distant metastases (Table 2).

Table 2. Main metastatic sites for the most common tumours in small animals.

Cancer	Species	Site of metastasis
Haemangiosarcoma	Dog	Liver, lungs, kidneys, omentum, eye, central nervous system
Osteosarcoma	Dog	Lungs, bone
Oral squamous cell carcinoma	Cat, dog	Lymph nodes, lungs
Mammary cancer	Cat, dog	Lymph nodes, lungs, bone
Prostate cancer	Dog	Lymph nodes, bone, lungs
Transitional cell carcinoma of the bladder	Dog	Lymph nodes, lungs, bone
Mast cell tumour	Dog	Lymph nodes, liver, spleen
	Cat	Spleen, liver, bone marrow

Adapted from *Manual of Small Animal Internal Medicine* (Nelson, Couto; 1999).

AIMS

- To identify concomitant diseases and determine their clinical stage.
- To differentiate between inflammation and malignancy.
- To identify cell lineage.
- To determine clinical stage.
- To identify the presence of paraneoplastic syndromes.

STEPS IN THE DIAGNOSTIC WORKUP

- Location of mass or masses (and where possible, marking of their location on a drawing of the pet [Fig. 13]).
- Complete blood count, basic biochemistry profile, electrolyte panels, and complete urine analysis.
- Fine-needle aspiration biopsy (FNAB), or fine-needle capillary sampling (FNCS).
- Biopsy if FNAB/FNCS is not diagnostic.
- Imaging studies: radiographs (right lateral, left lateral, dorsoventral, ventrodorsal), ultrasound, computed tomography, magnetic resonance imaging, endoscopy (as appropriate).
- Biopsy of excised mass where appropriate.

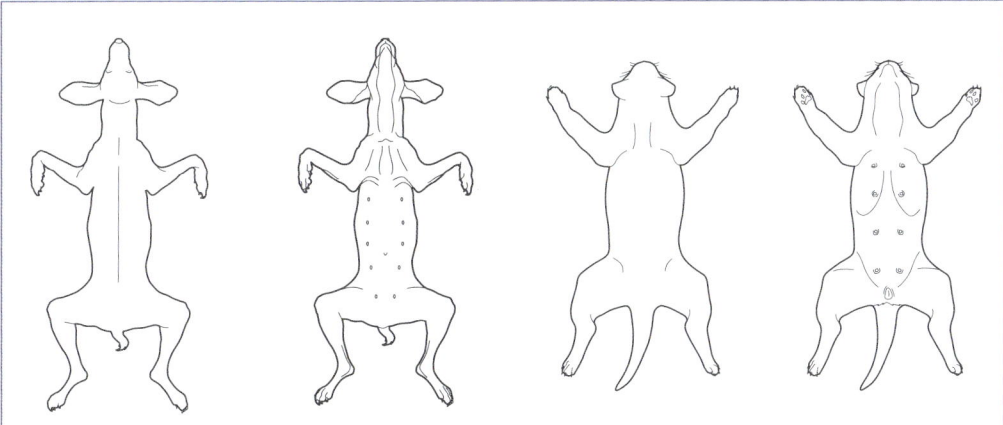

Figure 13. Diagrams for marking location of mass(es) in dogs (left) or cats (right).

3

Diagnostic procedures in veterinary oncology

In veterinary oncology, it is necessary to use practically all available diagnostic procedures in order to establish a definitive diagnosis, identify tumour stage, check for concomitant disease, decide on the best course of treatment, and establish a prognosis.

As mentioned in the previous chapter, patients should undergo a general evaluation prior to a specific oncological examination, as this can provide important information on when the tumour appeared, how it has progressed, and whether or not the patient has or has had other diseases (malignant or other).

Considering that most cases of cancer are seen in senior animals, the basic diagnostic workup should include a complete blood count, a basic biochemistry profile, electrolyte panels, and a complete urinalysis (with urine protein:creatinine ratio where appropriate).

Cytology

Introduction

Cytology is an essential diagnostic tool in cancer. The ease and speed with which both samples and results are obtained have positioned this tool as the diagnostic procedure of choice in many cases of suspected cancer.

The procedure involves examining the morphological features of isolated cells or clusters of cells to determine the origin of the lesion and differentiate between normal, inflammatory, hyperplastic, and neoplastic tissue. Cytological examinations can identify both the origin and degree of malignancy of a tumour, providing key information for establishing a prognosis, deciding on a treatment protocol, and monitoring disease course and response to treatment. Results can also serve to establish a diagnosis in certain cases (e.g. mast cell tumour [MCT], transmissible venereal tumour, and many types of lymphosarcoma [LSA]). In others, they provide sufficient information to raise suspicion of a tumour and guide the choice of subsequent tests. Finally, while results may not provide specific information on a tumour, they can rule out other diagnoses, facilitating the subsequent steps of the diagnostic workup.

It is important to recall that not all samples will be informative or of diagnostic aid. An estimated 40 % of samples collected in the veterinary practice are noninformative for reasons related to inadequate sample collection or processing (haemodilution, cell rupture) or technical limitations.

A reliable cytological diagnosis is only possible when samples containing a sufficient number of adequately stained intact cells arranged in a single layer are used.

Cytology should never replace biopsy as a diagnostic test.

Issuing a diagnosis based on cytological results only can result in a serious miscalculation of disease severity.

Cytology offers significant practical advantages. It is a simple, affordable test that carries few risks for the patient, and can be performed at any practice as it requires no special infrastructure or equipment. In addition, samples can be processed quickly in a highly versatile procedure that is applicable to practically all organs and structures:
- Cutaneous and subcutaneous masses.
- Lymph nodes.
- Solid organs: prostate, kidney, liver, spleen, lungs, pancreas, digestive tract.
- Bone marrow.
- Organ fluids:
  - Cerebrospinal fluid, synovial fluid, urine.
  - Effusions from body cavities: abdominal, pleural, or pericardial.
- Airway surface epithelial cells through nasal, tracheal, or bronchial lavages.
- Ear canal.
- Conjunctiva.
- Bone.
- Vagina.

Cytology, however, does not provide information on stromal characteristics or tissue architecture, which is crucial for establishing a definitive diagnosis in most cases. This is particularly true for tumours located in mammary tissue, where cytology does not provide the information required on degree of malignancy. Diagnosis in such cases must be confirmed by histopathology, which is essential for determining histological grade.

Cytology thus is a basic preliminary diagnostic tool and should be seen as a prior, complementary step to biopsy. Its results may help to guide the next steps of patient management, but, with very few exceptions, any definitive decisions must be made on the basis of histopathological findings.

Sample collection, slide preparation, and staining

Cytology is a very simple procedure. If the patient collaborates, sedation is not necessary, as the procedure is generally painless, even when samples need to be extracted from bones, abdominal organs, or mediastinal masses. Deep sedation is, however, required for the collection of lung samples. The risk of bleeding, infection, and tumour spread is minimal with cytology and should not be considered a limitation of the technique. While previous tests are not required for samples from external lesions, a reliable platelet count is needed when collecting samples from internal organs. In the absence of significant thrombocytopaenia, the risks of intracavitary bleeding are minimal, and with few exceptions (e.g. suspected disseminated intravascular coagulation), coagulation tests are not necessary. Ultrasound can be used to guide the collection of samples from internal organs.

Cytology samples can be collected using fine-needle capillary sampling (FNCS) or fine-needle aspiration biopsy (FNAB). Unlike FNAB, FNCS preserves cell integrity and is therefore the procedure of choice for tissues whose cells break easily (e.g. lymph nodes). The latter technique is also recommended for highly vascular lesions, as it minimises the risk of blood contamination.

By contrast, FNAB is recommended for minimally exfoliative lesions, as it preserves a higher cell content. This technique, however, offers few other advantages in this setting, positioning fine-needle capillary sampling as the first-line procedure in most cases.

The choice of needle in FNCS is determined by the size, location, and depth of the lesion, although a 22- to 25-gauge needle is generally sufficient. To perform the procedure, insert the needle into the lesion and redirect it several times without applying suction. These redirection movements should be rapid (three per second) and the needle inserted to a depth of at least 1.5 cm where possible.

In the case of FNAB, 5- to 10-cc syringes and 20- to 23-gauge needles are used. The aim in FNAB is to collect sufficient material without it passing through the cone of the needle. Suction should be applied once the needle is inserted in the lesion and released before it is withdrawn.

Diagnostic yield can be improved by taking several samples from the same lesion. Tumours, and large tumours in particular, are heterogeneous lesions and therefore FNAB results may vary depending on the needle insertion point. Peripheral areas should be prioritised as they are more likely than central areas to contain necrotic material. Ulcerated areas should also be avoided, as they tend to contain inflammatory material. Scraping or impression can be used to collect sample in such cases, but the likelihood of obtaining an informative sample is very low.

Samples from the respiratory tract are generally collected using nasal, tracheobronchial, or bronchoalveolar lavage techniques. Lavage fluid is processed in a similar way to organ fluid.

The first step is to prepare and fix the smear immediately. This is done by spreading the sample on a slide in a single layer of cells that can be uniformly dyed. To do this, place the material at one edge of the slide and spread it across evenly using the squash technique (Fig. 1). If the material is highly contaminated with blood, it can be prepared as a blood smear.

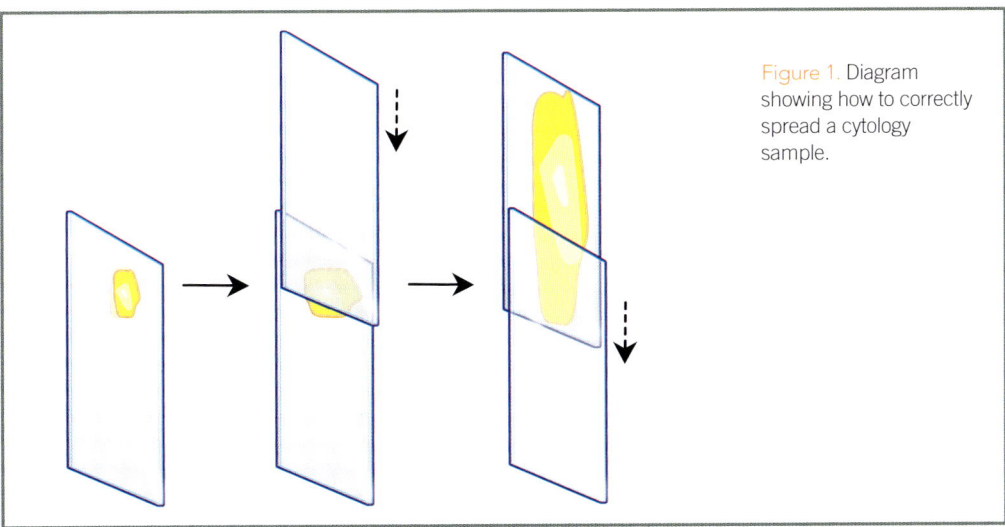

Figure 1. Diagram showing how to correctly spread a cytology sample.

Lavage or body fluid cytology samples must be processed immediately to prevent cell degeneration. Collection in EDTA tubes preserves cell morphology, while cytocentrifugation increases the concentration of cells, resulting in significantly improved quality.

Romanowsky stains (Giemsa, May–Grünwald–Giemsa, and rapid stains) are the most widely used stains in cytology, as they generally offer excellent cytoplasmic and adequate nuclear detail. Rapid stains are adequate for a preliminary evaluation, but they provide less detail.

Cell interpretation protocol

Cytology results should be interpreted as follows:
- **Using a low-magnification (10x) objective lens**, check that the sample has been correctly spread across the slide and that there are enough intact, properly stained cells. Discard any broken cells and choose the most representative slides.
  - Cytological diagnosis will not be possible if the above basic requirements are not met.
  - Evaluate the number, type, and distribution of cells in the sample and choose the most suitable areas for diagnosis (i.e. those containing a single layer of correctly stained cells).
- **Using a medium objective lens (40x)**, examine the selected areas to identify the predominant cell type(s), and depending on their morphology, classify them as inflammatory or tissue-type.
  - If they are tissue-type cells, establish their origin and check for cytological features of malignancy.

- **Using the higher-magnification objective lens (100× with immersion oil),**
  - examine the cells in greater detail to confirm their origin and grade of malignancy. In many cases, a 40× lens will be sufficient.
  - Check for microorganisms.

Biopsy

Biopsy is the procedure of choice for establishing a definitive diagnosis, determining the biological behaviour and malignancy of a tumour, and guiding decisions on surgical treatment.

It should be performed when:
1. The cytology results are inconclusive.
2. The type and extent of treatment (radiation therapy, chemotherapy, or surgery) could be altered by identification of tumour type or grade.
3. The results could change the owner's willingness to continue treatment.

Biopsy samples are also required for immunohistochemical staining, which is a valuable tool for establishing diagnosis and assessing alternative treatments. There are several types of biopsy procedures.

- **Thick-needle biopsy.** This is performed using 14-gauge needles (Tru-Cut) and it provides soft tissue samples of approximately 1 mm in thickness and 1–1.5 cm in length. It is indicated for palpable masses located in internal organs (kidneys, liver, or prostate), and requires deep sedation or general anaesthesia.
- **Punch biopsy.** This provides a deep, narrow specimen (2–8 mm). It is used to collect samples from accessible masses (e.g. in the skin, oral cavity, perianal area) or from body cavities (e.g. liver biopsy during a laparotomy).
- **Incisional biopsy.** This is used when the above techniques (including cytology) do not provide a diagnosis. It is the procedure of choice for ulcerated or

necrotic tumours, as it achieves larger samples that can be used to evaluate representative areas of the tumour. Incisional biopsy requires sterile surgical preparation and involves the extraction of part of the lesion for subsequent examination.
- **Excisional biopsy.** This technique is used for both diagnostic and therapeutic purposes, as it consists of completely excising the mass, together with margins of healthy tissue (Fig. 2).
- **Other.** Biopsy of intra-abdominal, bone, or intrathoracic lesions requires the use of additional techniques, such as endoscopy, ultrasound, computerised tomography (CT), and magnetic resonance imaging (MRI).

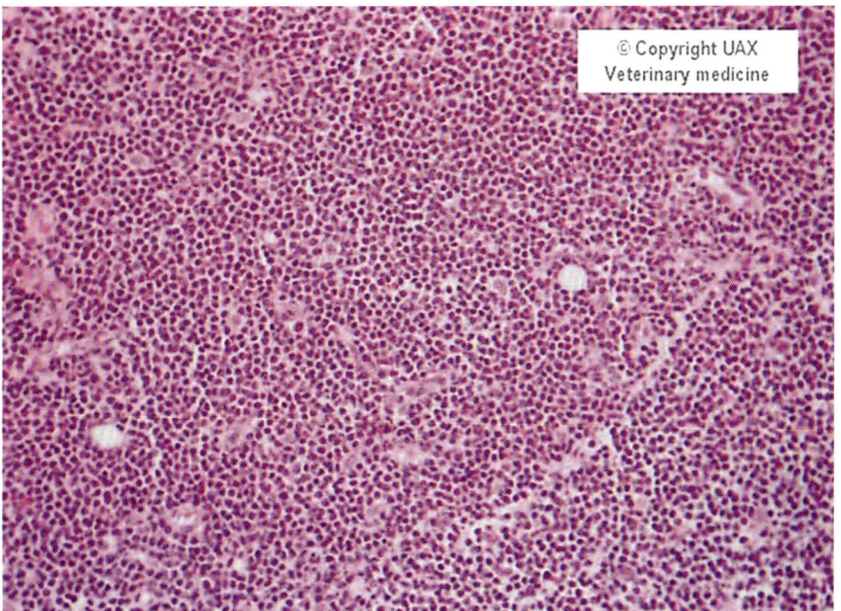

Figure 2. Biopsy sample from a lymph node showing findings consistent with lymphoma. *Image courtesy of Fernando Vázquez, Veterinary Teaching Hospital, Alfonso X El Sabio University.*

Blood and bone marrow smears

Blood smears are an essential part of the diagnostic workup as most animals with cancer are elderly and may have concomitant diseases or blood alterations caused by the tumour (anaemia, polycythaemia, thrombocytopaenia, bone marrow metastases).

An **elevated red blood cell (RBC) count** (polycythaemia) rarely indicates the presence of a tumour. The main causes of erythrocytosis are dehydration, cardiorespiratory disorders, Cushing's syndrome, corticosteroid therapy, and polycythaemia vera. **Anaemia** is common in oncological patients and it can be regenerative (haemorrhage-associated, immune-mediated haemolytic anaemia) or nonregenerative (associated with bone marrow disease) (see Appendix I).

A persistent or unexplained increase in a patient's **white blood cell** (WBC) count may indicate the presence of leukaemia or bone marrow invasion by a lymphoma (stage V disease). Counts above 50,000 WBCs in dogs and above 35,000 in cats are highly suggestive of leukaemia and are normally accompanied by altered RBC and platelet counts. Detection of leukocytosis and/or the presence of abnormal WBC forms in a smear calls for a bone marrow biopsy to categorise the disease, decide on the course of treatment, and establish a prognosis. Lymphoid leukaemia is the most common type of leukaemia and includes acute lymphoblastic leukaemia and chronic lymphocytic leukaemia. Acute lymphoblastic leukaemia tends to affect young or middle-aged animals. It runs an acute or hyperacute course and is characterised by mild generalised lymphadenopathy, splenomegaly, and, on occasions, fever. Chronic lymphocytic leukaemia affects elderly animals. It runs an insidious course and is diagnosed after excluding all other causes of lymphocytosis.

Thrombocytopaenia may be observed in cancer. A blood smear can confirm this condition and rule out that it is not due to platelet clumping.

A **bone marrow study** is indicated in patients with anaemia, persistent leukopaenia, persistent thrombocytopaenia, or suspected myelophthisis or myelodysplasia. The results are presented as the percentage of cells in each population. In normal conditions, less than 2 % of nucleated bone marrow cells are plasma cells. Percentages in excess of 3 % should raise suspicion of immunostimulation. An increase in plasma cells can be caused by an infectious disease (e.g. ehrlichiosis) or multiple myeloma (MM). Low proportions of mast cells in bone marrow are a normal finding. High counts or abnormal forms may indicate metastasis from an MCT. In normal conditions, 15–20 % of the cell population is composed of mature lymphocytes. Rates >30 % should raise suspicion of a lymphoid tumour. Metastases from other types of tumours, such as carcinomas, are possible but are less common.

Flow cytometry and PCR for antigen receptor rearrangements

Flow cytometry involves the use of laser to identify membrane or intracellular molecules through specific fluorescent antibodies. The procedure is generally used to identify cluster of differentiation (CD) antigens (Table 1).

In oncology, flow cytometry is particularly useful for classifying lymphoproliferative and histiocytic disorders.

The importance of immunophenotyping in canine lymphoma

There is evidence that classifying lymphoma using cell markers or flow cytometry has prognostic value. B-cell lymphomas are the most common form of lymphoma in dogs and have a better prognosis than their T-cell counterparts. Some authors have described a mean survival of 389 days for B-cell lymphomas compared with 159 days for T-cell lymphomas. However, these data are mainly applicable to the multicentric form of lymphoma, as little information has been published on the use of cell markers or flow cytometry to classify extranodal variants.

Flow cytometry

Flow cytometry is increasingly being used in veterinary medicine. It consists of labelling cells with antibodies that bind to cell-surface or intracellular receptors (CD, Table 1). These cells are then passed through a tube where they are exposed to laser light. Different receptors capture the amount and polarisation of scattered light and the fluorescence emitted by the antibodies used to label the cells (Fig. 3). The results are shown in graph format and as numbers (Fig. 4). They show information on the size of cells, their internal complexity, and the antibodies used.

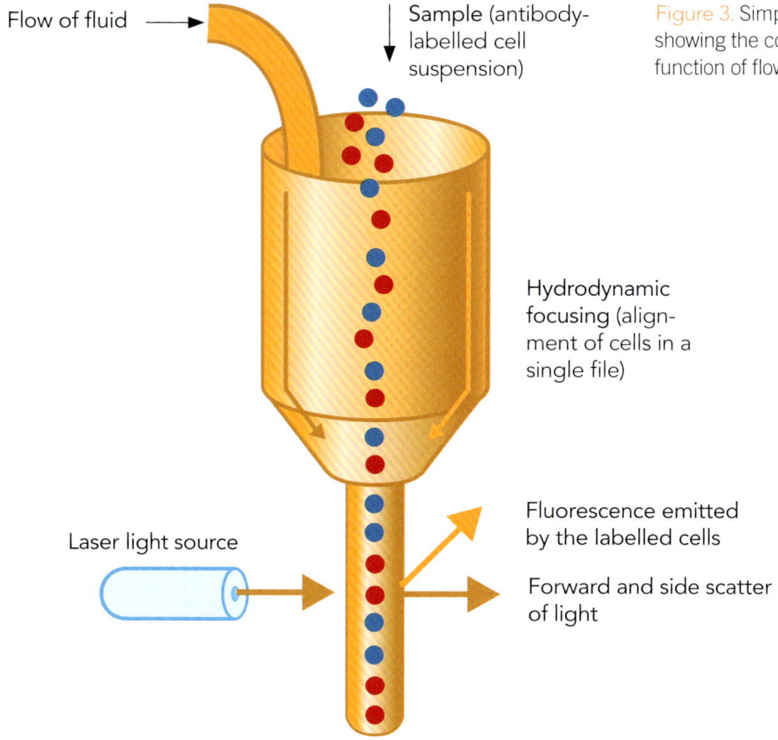

Flow of fluid
Sample (antibody-labelled cell suspension)
Hydrodynamic focusing (alignment of cells in a single file)
Laser light source
Fluorescence emitted by the labelled cells
Forward and side scatter of light

Figure 3. Simplified diagram showing the components and function of flow cytometry.

A06 m CD3 FITC-r CD8 PE
Gate: (R1 in all)
Q6-UL
0.1%
Q6-UR
81.7%
Q6-LL
16.4%
Q6-LR
1.8%
PE-H
FITC-H

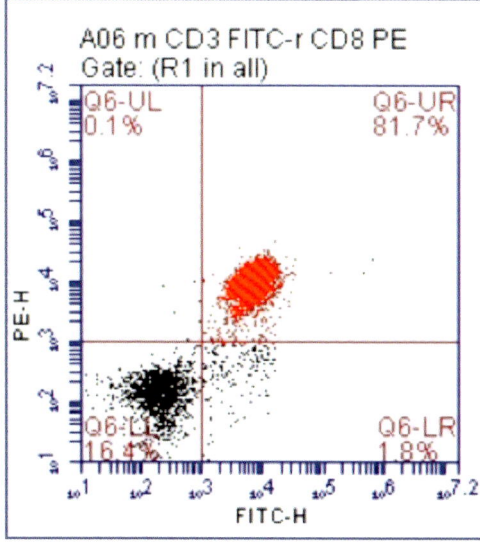

Figure 4. Graph showing flow cytometry results for a lymph node aspirate from a patient with a suspected lymphoma. $CD3^+$ and $CD8^+$ cells are shown on the horizontal and vertical axes, respectively. The upper right quadrant is positive for both markers while the lower left quadrant is negative. Most cells are recognised as $CD8^+$ T cells.

Flow cytometry requirements:
- Samples must be collected before initiation of any medical treatment to avoid alterations to the neoplastic lymphocyte population, as, unlike PARR (see next), cytometry identifies population groups rather than clonal populations.
- The cells must be suspended in a solution; tissue fragments or cytological smears should therefore not be submitted to the laboratory. The following samples are ideal for use in flow cytometry:
  - Liquid samples: pleural or peritoneal effusions and cerebrospinal fluid.
  - Blood samples collected in EDTA tubes when there are high numbers of circulating neoplastic cells (stage IV LSA) or when lymphoid or myeloid leukaemia is suspected.
  - Fine-needle aspiration can be used to collect tissue samples. The addition of a small amount of serum (bovine or patient) to the saline solution will help to preserve the tissue cells during transport to the laboratory.
- Sufficient numbers of viable cells are necessary. In general, when samples are taken from a lymph node, the suspension should have a cloudy white colour.
- Samples must be transported rapidly under refrigeration and analysed within 3 days of collection. They should never be frozen as this can destroy the cells.

Table 1. List of most widely used antigens in flow cytometry immunophenotyping of lymphoma together with the cells they express.

Marker	Cell expression
CD45	All leukocytes
CD18	All leukocytes (more in lymphocytes)
CD21	Mature B cells
CD79a	B cells in all stages
CD5	T cells
CD3	T cells
CD4	T helper cells and neutrophils
CD8	Cytotoxic T cells
CD14	Monocytes
CD34	Hematopoietic blasts
MHC II	Antigen-presenting cells
CD1a	Histiocytic (dendritic) cells
CD11c	Histiocytic cells. Present in Langerhans/dendritic cells and interstitial cells
CD11d	Histiocytic cells with macrophage differentiation

Uses of immunophenotyping in lymphoma:
1. **Identification of cell type.** Immunophenotyping can identify the different populations of cells in a sample.
2. **Estimation of tumour maturity status.**
   a. Precursor lymphoid and myeloid cells express CD34. When there are neoplastic cells in the bone marrow or blood, CD34 helps to distinguish between acute leukaemia (CD3$^+$) and stage V lymphoma or lymphoproliferative disease (CD3$^-$). The distinction between stage V lymphoma and chronic leukaemia is more complicated and must be based mainly on clinical findings. Aberrant expression of CD34 may also be observed in certain lymphomas.
   b. CD21 and CD79a are used to distinguish between mature (CD21$^+$CD79a$^+$) and immature B cells (CD21$^-$CD79a$^+$).
   c. Immature T cells in the thymic cortex are double-negative (CD4$^-$CD8$^-$) but change to double-positive when they mature (CD4$^+$CD8$^+$). By interacting with antigen-presenting cells in the thymus, they differentiate into T helper (CD4$^+$CD8$^-$) or cytotoxic (CD4$^-$CD8$^+$) cells and migrate towards secondary lymphoid organs, blood, and bone marrow. This maturation process is useful for distinguishing between mediastinal lymphoma, which tends to display clonal expansion of cells with a specific immunophenotype, and thymoma, which tends to display a high number of CD4$^+$ and CD8$^+$ cells.
3. **Detection of abnormal patterns.** An abnormal immunophenotype profile indicates qualitative or quantitative alterations in antigen expression in neoplastic lymphoid cells. It is useful for detecting minimal residual disease and, in some cases, for establishing a prognosis. Abnormal patterns do not indicate a worse prognosis (Table 2). The most common abnormal immunophenotype profiles in lymphoma are B and T cell–antigen coexpression (CD3$^+$CD79$^+$ and CD3$^+$CD21$^+$), CD34 expression, CD4 and CD8 coexpression in T lymphocytes, and loss of leukocyte antigens, such as CD45 and CD18.

Table 2. **Examples of abnormal surface marker expression and associated prognosis.**

Abnormal pattern	Prognosis
Low expression of MHC II in B-cell lymphoma	Higher mortality and shorter time to recurrence
Loss of CD45 in T-zone lymphoma	CD45 expression is associated with much shorter survival
Loss of CD45 in CD4$^+$ T-cell lymphoma	Indolent clinical course
Decreased MHC II expression in CD4$^+$ T-cell lymphoma	Aggressive clinical course

4. **Staging and detection of minimal residual disease.** Flow cytometry helps to assess the extent of disease by identifying neoplastic peripheral blood, bone marrow, liver, and spleen cells. Detection of lymphocytes displaying an abnormal pattern helps to identify the presence of tumour-reactive lymphocytes in a normal lymphocyte population, enabling thus early diagnosis. In large B-cell lymphoma, populations of large B cells >3 % in bone marrow have been linked to shorter survival (115 vs 322 days) and faster disease progression (69 vs 149 days) than populations <3 %.

Cell proliferation markers such as Ki67 are also of some value for predicting outcomes in dogs with high-grade B-cell lymphoma. Patients with a Ki67 expression of less than 20.1 % in neoplastic cells have been found to survive for longer than those with higher expression levels.

The main disadvantages of flow cytometry are the need for fresh samples with sufficient cell numbers, the high cost of antibodies and dedicated equipment, and the need for expert interpretation of results.

PCR for antigen receptor rearrangements

PCR for antigen receptor rearrangements (PARR) is a molecular diagnostic tool that works on the basic principle that most lymphocytes in lymphoproliferative diseases belong to the same clone, and accordingly, the DNA encoding the membrane receptors expressed on B or T cells will be homogeneous throughout the neoplastic population (monoclonal expansion). In normal circumstances, B- and T-cell receptors are as varied as the antigens they recognise. Accordingly, this variety will be reflected by the expansion profile of the DNA encoding these receptors (polyclonal expansion) in the PARR results.

Unlike cytometry, PARR can be used to analyse formalin-fixed tissue samples, frozen samples, cytology samples, and fluid samples.

Its main application is to differentiate between reactive and neoplastic lymphoid proliferations when cytology or histology tests are inconclusive. This technique should not be used in isolation for immunophenotyping, as it has a high rate of false positives and negatives.

It should also not be used as a screening tool in healthy patients, as it has been found to detect just 75 % of confirmed cases of canine lymphoma in dogs and 65 % in cats. Its respective sensitivity and specificity rates are 94 % and 75 % for dogs and 65 % and 90 % for cats.

PARR results can be interpreted as follows:
1. Monoclonal or biclonal B-cell or T-cell expansion (with polyclonal expansion of the other population) is consistent with B-cell or T-cell lymphoma.
2. Polyclonal B- and T-cell expansion is consistent with the presence of normal or hyperplastic lymphoid tissue.

As mentioned, PARR can produce false-positive and false-negative results:
1. False negatives
   a. Inadequate primer coverage (insufficient primer sets to cover the target genes). This is uncommon but possible.
   b. Mutations at primer binding sites due to somatic hypermutation of B cells.
   c. Excessive polyclonal background, either because the lymphoma arose in a previously reactive lymph node or because the tumour contains lymphocytes induced by an inflammatory response.
2. False positives (uncommon)
   a. Clonal expansion in response to antigen stimulation. This has been observed in histiocytoma and is suspected to occur in ehrlichiosis and leishmaniosis.
   b. Unspecific amplification due to technical issues.

Considering the above limitations, PARR results must be integrated with clinical, morphological, and/or immunophenotypic findings.

Main advantages of PARR:
- Ability to analyse a wide variety of samples, including those collected a long time ago.
- Minimally invasive, as it can be used to analyse aspirates collected for cytology.
- Ability to detect a cloned cell among 100 normal cells.
- Relatively affordable price compared with other tests.

Main disadvantages of PARR:
- Need for species-specific primers.
- Need for personnel with expertise and experience in genetics.

Although much remains to be done to refine the criteria guiding the use of PARR as a therapeutic and prognostic tool, veterinary surgeons need to be familiar with the use, possibilities, and limitations of new techniques such as this in order to harness their full potential.

Diagnostic imaging in veterinary oncology

Diagnostic imaging has a crucial role in veterinary oncology, and the techniques available have a wide range of applications, from diagnosis through to staging. Diagnostic imaging techniques are also essential for planning certain treatments, such as surgery or radiation therapy.

The most common techniques used in veterinary oncology are radiography, ultrasound, CT, and MRI.

The choice of one or more of these techniques depends on several factors:
- Type of tumour being investigated. Chest radiography, for example, is essential for monitoring malignant mammary tumours, while CT or MRI is essential for planning surgery in injection-site sarcomas.
- Geographic distribution of technology (access to practices and owners).
- Affordability for owners. A veterinary surgeon should never take it for granted that an owner can afford a test. Owners should always be informed about the best diagnostic options available and given the opportunity to weigh up the options and decide what to do.
- Sensitivity and specificity rates (likelihood of false positives and negatives) help to indicate the reliability of different tests. Sensitivity refers to the likelihood of a positive result when a patient has a given disease, whereas specificity refers to the likelihood of a negative result when the patient does not have the disease.

Thankfully, owners are increasingly sensitive to the well-being of their pets and more and more demanding when it comes to diagnostic accuracy and treatment effectiveness. Imaging techniques have therefore become part of many routine diagnostic workups, resulting in greater overall treatment success.

Apart from their value as diagnostic and staging tools, imaging techniques also have an important role in monitoring disease course, detecting new lesions, and assessing response to treatment over time.

Radiography

Radiography is the most widely accessible and affordable imaging technique in veterinary medicine, and image quality on the whole has greatly improved thanks to advances in digital radiography.

Several views are generally required to overcome the problems associated with overlapping structures or artefacts, as X-rays provide 2-dimensional images of 3-dimensional body structures. Radiography has moderate sensitivity, and specificity is high only when it is used to study bone lesions.

Its main indication in veterinary oncology is the evaluation of lung metastases from solid tumours. It is also useful for detecting bone lesions and evaluating enlarged thoracic lymph nodes, and while it can reveal organomegaly in the abdomen, it cannot identify the cause.

Radiography also has a role in preoperative studies as most patients with cancer are geriatric and may have cardiorespiratory disorders that complicate the use of anaesthesia.

More advanced imaging techniques are needed to identify lung lesions <5 mm in diameter or to distinguish tumours from inflammatory lesions.

Applications of radiography by location:
- **Chest radiography.** Used to visualise thoracic masses, lymphadenopathies, and metastases >5 mm in diameter. It is also useful for investigating pleural involvement (Figs. 5 and 6). Characteristics:

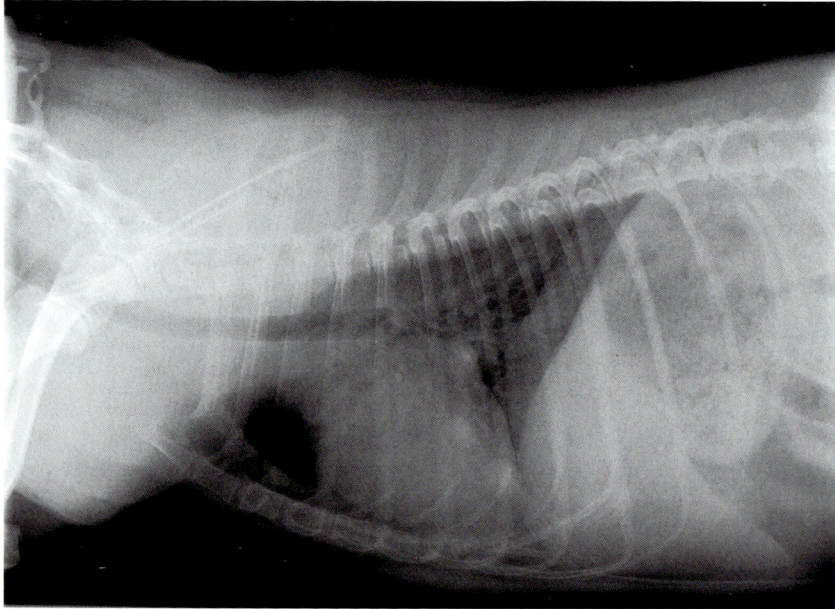

Figure 5. X-ray of a pulmonary metastasis with a nodular pattern in a dog.

- At least two (but preferably three) projections are needed (right lateral and left lateral [Fig. 7] and ventrodorsal or dorsoventral [Fig. 8]).
- These projections should form part of any preoperative study.
- Detection of an image consistent with malignancy calls for additional investigation by CT to confirm the presence and number of lesions and their exact location (pleura, lungs, mediastinum).

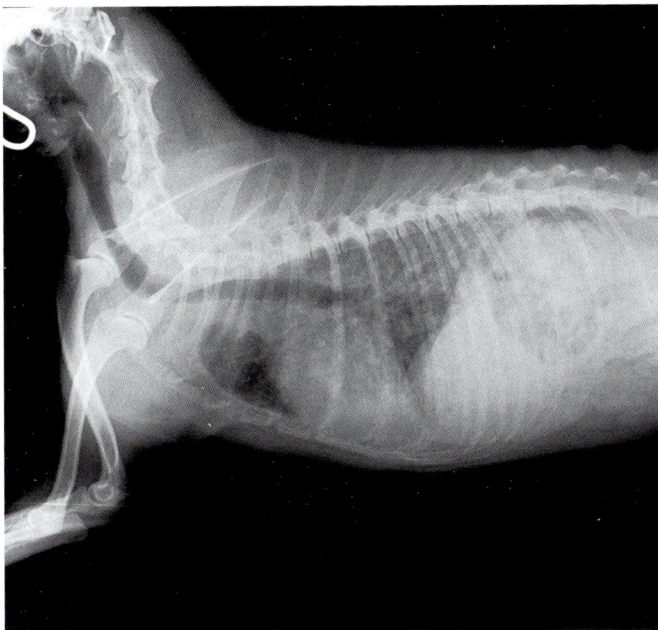

Figure 6. X-ray of a pulmonary metastasis with a miliary pattern.

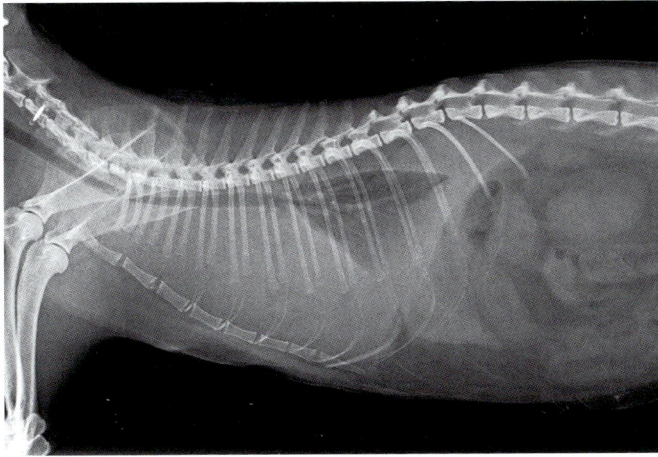

Figure 7. Lateral view in a cat with pleural effusion.

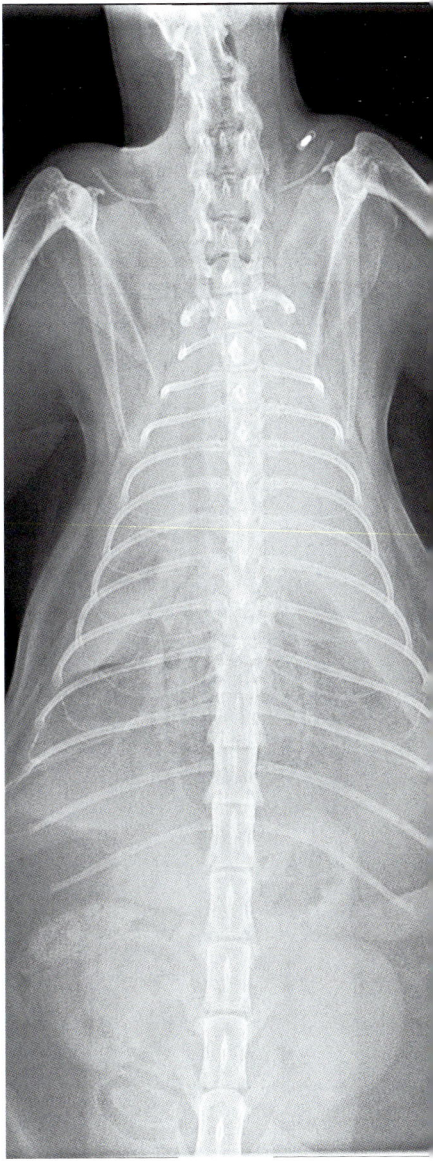

Figure 8. Ventrodorsal view of the cat in Figure 7.

MOST COMMON LUNG PATTERNS

- **Interstitial**

  Unstructured/linear:
  - Diffuse: technical error, elderly animals, tumours (lymphosarcoma, haemangiosarcoma), pneumonia.
  - Localised: partial lung collapse, contusion, haemorrhage, foreign body.

  Nodular: tumour (primary, metastasis), granuloma, abscess, bulla.

- **Bronchial:** bronchitis, bronchiectasis.
- **Alveolar**

  Generalised: pneumonia, oedema.

  Focal/multifocal: pneumonia, oedema, haemorrhage.
- **Vascular**

- **Abdominal radiography.** Abdominal X-rays provide little information in oncology. Although they show organ and lymph node enlargement (Fig. 9), additional imaging tests, such as ultrasound and even CT and RMI, are needed to detect the cause.
  - Two projections (lateral and ventrodorsal) are required.
  - They can identify organ displacement possibly caused by an intra-abdominal mass.

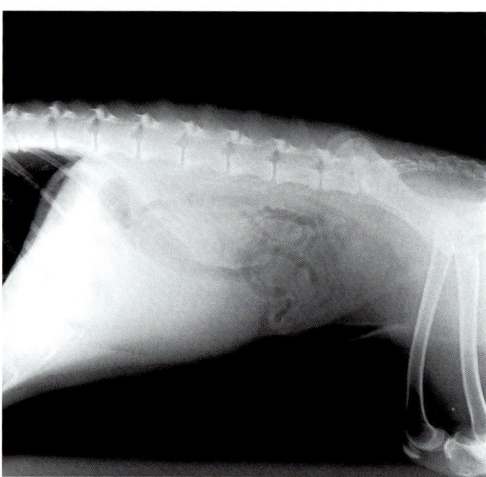

Figure 9. Abdominal X-ray showing hepatomegaly in an animal diagnosed with hepatic carcinoma. Note the dorsocaudal displacement of the organs.

- **Bone radiography.** Bone X-rays have high sensitivity and specificity for both osteophytic and proliferative skeletal lesions.
  - Two projections are also necessary in this case.
  - Bilateral joint involvement is very rare in primary bone tumours and should raise suspicion of a joint tumour or a lesion in the adjacent soft tissues involving the bone.

- Although bone X-rays clearly identify the presence and size of a lesion and the degree of bone destruction, they cannot identify the type of tumour involved. This must be done by ultrasound-guided biopsy or fine-needle aspiration aimed at identifying "windows" of soft tissue providing access to the lesion (Fig. 10).
- **Contrast radiography.** This technique has low sensitivity and has now largely been replaced by ultrasound. It is used to investigate:
  - The digestive tract, where luminal narrowing or obstructions can indicate a possible tumour. Barium is the most common contrast agent used in this case, although iodine agents are recommended when perforation or complete obstruction is suspected.
  - The bladder, where the combined use of iodine and air can show growths or irregularities in the bladder wall.

Ultrasound

Ultrasound is more costly than radiography. It has high sensitivity but low to moderate specificity as it often cannot differentiate between benign and malignant lesions. (A splenic haematoma, for example, can resemble haemangiosarcoma [HSA] on ultrasound.) Specialist knowledge is also needed for test performance and interpretation.

Finally, ultrasound is the imaging method of choice for diagnosing intra-abdominal tumours, as it normally shows the exact location of the tumour (Fig. 11). It is also very useful for evaluating masses in pleural, pericardial, or peritoneal effusions and for guiding the collection of fluid samples (Fig. 12).

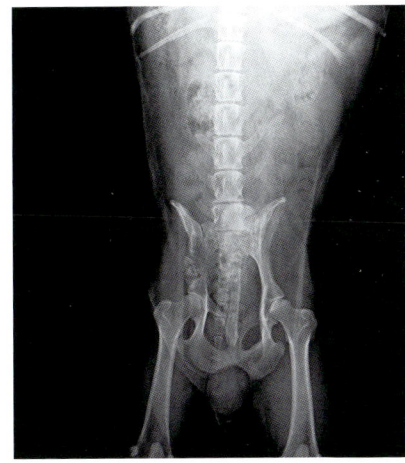

Figure 10. X-ray showing lytic and proliferative lesions in the ilium of a dog subsequently diagnosed with haemangiosarcoma by biopsy.

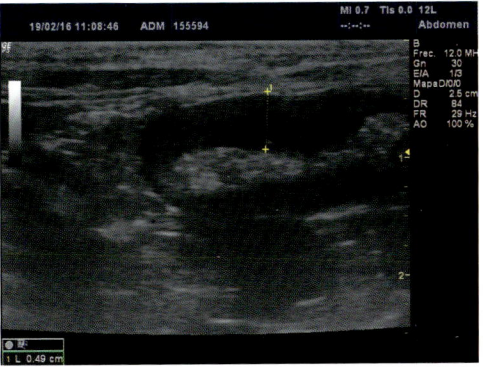

Figure 11. Abdominal ultrasound of a cat showing thickened and altered layers of the intestinal wall. Cytology confirmed the diagnosis of mast cell tumour.

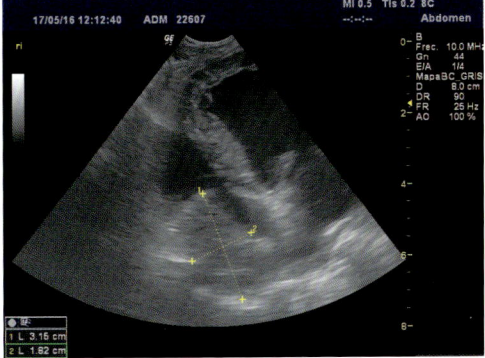

Figure 12. Splenic mass associated with haemoperitoneum.

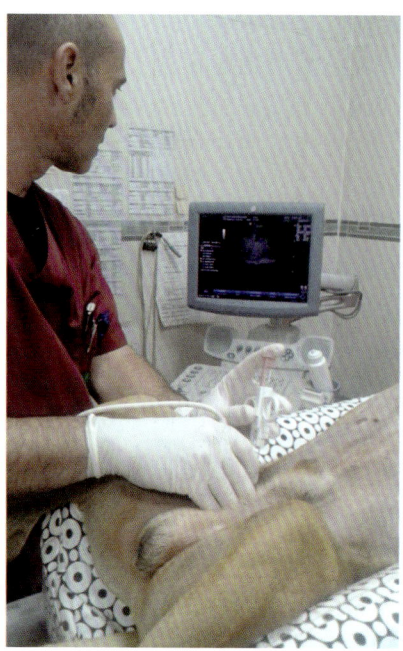

Figure 13. Ultrasound-guided prostate biopsy.

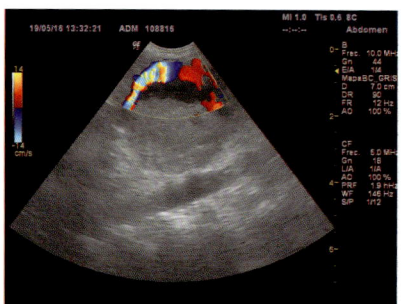

Figure 14. Vascularity of a splenic mass.

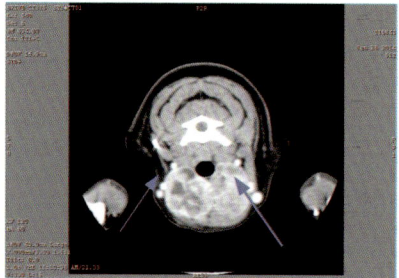

Figure 15. CT image showing a bilateral thyroid mass. Note the high uptake of contrast material.

Ultrasound is an essential tool for guiding the collection of biological samples (cytology, biopsy) from lesions located in body cavities or in deeper parts of the body, such as muscle, bone, and thyroid glands (Fig. 13).

It also has a role in identifying enlarged lymph nodes and distant metastases, and in the case of Doppler imaging, evaluating lesion vascularity (Fig. 14).

Ultrasound is an essential staging tool for tumours such as lymphoma, MCT, mammary tumours, HSA, and apocrine gland adenosarcoma of anal sac origin.

Computed tomography

Computed tomography is an advanced imaging technique based on X-rays. It is a costly procedure, but it has high sensitivity and specificity, as it renders 3-dimensional pictures that eliminate the problem of overlapping structures seen on conventional X-rays. It also offers superior greyscale resolution. Its performance and interpretation require specialist knowledge.

Iodine-based contrast agents are typically used in CT scanning, as they provide better soft-tissue definition. As tumours tend to take up much more iodine contrast than soft tissue, CT scans help to detect neoplasms and enlarged lymph nodes by showing a greater contrast between these structures and adjacent tissue (Fig. 15).

Computed tomography is also a useful tool for planning aggressive surgery in tumours that require wide margins (e.g. injection-site sarcomas). It can also be used to evaluate the vascularity of the mass and guide the collection of biopsy or cytology samples in locations that are difficult to reach.
Main indications of CT:
- Diagnosis of oral or nasal masses and definition of margins.
- Evaluation of thoracic masses and lung metastases with a diameter <5 mm.
- Surgical planning for limb-sparing surgery in animals with limb tumours (Fig. 16).
- Determination of true margins and operability in highly invasive tumours, such as infiltrative lipomas, soft-tissue sarcomas, and apocrine gland adenocarcinoma of the anal sac (Figs. 17 and 18).
- Planning of radiation therapy (Fig. 19).
- Detection of enlarged lymph nodes, such as in cases of metastasis to the iliac nodes in apocrine gland adenocarcinoma of the anal sac (Fig. 20). In this case, CT is essential.
- Although MRI is preferable, CT is also quite useful for evaluating intracranial masses (Fig. 21).
- Diagnosis of bone or joint tumours.

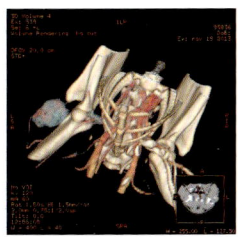

Figure 16. 3-Dimensional reconstruction showing the vascularity of a sarcoma in the shoulder area.

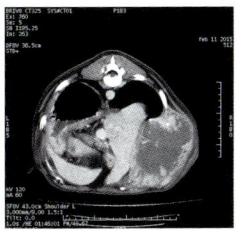

Figure 17. CT scan to evaluate a subcutaneous mass subsequently diagnosed as haemangiosarcoma of a rib.

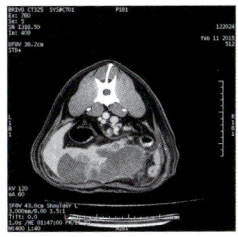

Figure 18. CT image from same patient as above but in addition showing a splenic lesion.

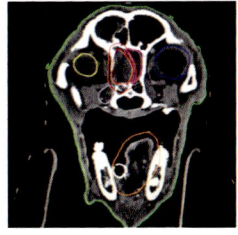

Figure 19. CT planning of radiation therapy to treat a meningioma. *Image courtesy of Dr Víctor Domingo, Ciovet.*

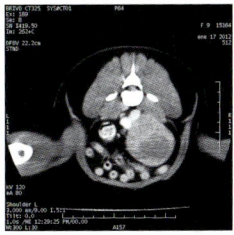

Figure 20. Abdominal CT scan showing regional lymph node enlargement in a patient with apocrine gland carcinoma of the anal sac.

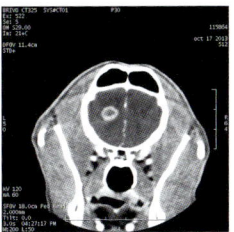

Figure 21. CT scan of a dog showing an intracranial nodular pattern consistent with a tumour.

Magnetic resonance imaging

Magnetic resonance imaging is a sophisticated diagnostic technique with limited availability and high equipment, installation, and maintenance costs. Like ultrasound and CT, its performance and interpretation require specialist knowledge.

It is ideal for diagnosing and monitoring tumours in the central nervous system, spine, and muscle, and provides greater definition than CT for soft-tissue tumours. However, MRI is not indicated for the diagnosis of bone tumours or primary or metastatic lung tumours.

In addition, examination times are relatively long and require general anaesthesia.

As with CT, the use of contrast agents enhances visibility and definition.

Endoscopy

Gastrointestinal endoscopy

In dogs and cats, 70 % percent of gastrointestinal tumours are located in the oral cavity; the rest are located in the large intestine (20 %) and the stomach (10 %). Tumours of the small intestine have a low incidence in dogs, but are more common in cats. Oesophageal cancer is rare.

Many gastrointestinal tumours can be identified by endoscopic examination of the gastrointestinal tract with the collection of biopsies. The main advantage of gastrointestinal endoscopy is that it can be used to directly visualise the digestive tract, identify the location and extent of tumours and lesions, and collect biopsies for subsequent histopathological examination. It is also very useful for mucosal lesions (epithelial or lymphoproliferative tumours), but conventional surgery and biopsy of the full thickness of the digestive wall are sometimes necessary for deeper lesions, such as leiomyomas, leiomyosarcomas, and stromal tumours.

Oesophageal tumours

Endoscopic examination of the oesophagus is the technique of choice for the identification of oesophageal tumours. In patients with tumours involving muscle, accurate diagnosis requires the collection of several biopsies from the same site to ensure sufficient penetration into the muscle layer of the oesophagus.

Primary oesophageal tumours are uncommon and include carcinomas, muscle tumours, osteosarcomas, and sarcomas secondary to *Spirocerca lupi* infestation.

Macroscopically, carcinomas (squamous cell carcinoma, glandular carcinoma, and neuroendocrine carcinoma) appear as an isolated mass and occur in the cervical or thoracic oesophagus. Leiomyomas, leiomyosarcomas, and stromal tumours are more frequently located in the area near the gastroesophageal sphincter.

Osteosarcomas and sarcomas associated with *Spirocerca lupi* infestation are more common in the thoracic oesophagus.

There have also been reports of secondary oesophageal tumours due to metastases from thyroid carcinomas, gastric carcinomas, and multicentric lymphomas (Fig. 22). These secondary tumours do not appear to have a predilection for any specific location.

Gastric tumours

Endoscopic examination is very useful for analysing gastric tumours involving the mucosa, as it serves to determine the exact location and extent of the tumour and to collect biopsy specimens from different areas.

The most common primary gastric masses are polyps and adenomas, tumours invading the muscle layer, lymphoproliferative tumours, and gastric carcinoma.

Gastric polyps (non-neoplastic polyps and true adenomas) present as solitary or multiple lesions with a pedunculated appearance that are typically located in the pyloric antrum (Fig. 23). They are largely asymptomatic and tend to be found incidentally. Non-neoplastic or inflammatory polyps can only be distinguished from true **adenomas** by biopsy.

Tumours affecting the **muscle layer** are mainly located in the area of the pyloric antrum, the pyloric sphincter, or in the first portions of the duodenum. They have also been observed as an extension of an oesophageal muscle tumour in the region of the gastroesophageal sphincter or cardia (Fig. 24).

Lymphoproliferative tumours (gastric LSA) can occur in any part of the stomach, although they are most frequently located in the pyloric antrum or the first portions of the duodenum. They can be multifocal (affecting the stomach, small intestine, and colon).

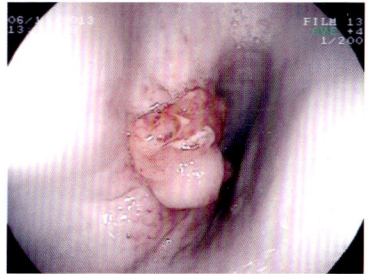

Figure 22. Endoscopic image of a lymphosarcoma in the thoracic oesophagus (oesophageal tumour secondary to multicentric lymphoma).

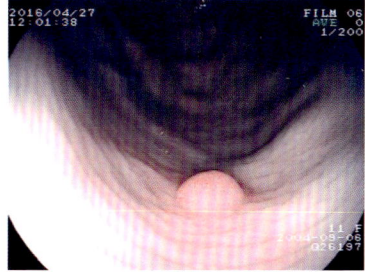

Figure 23. Endoscopic image of an adenoma in the pyloric antrum.

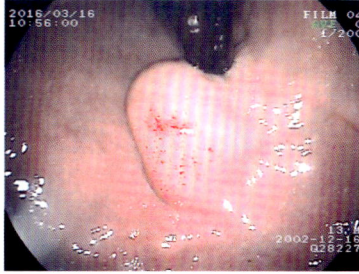

Figure 24. Endoscopic image of a leiomyosarcoma in the gastric fundus (gastroesophageal sphincter region or cardia).

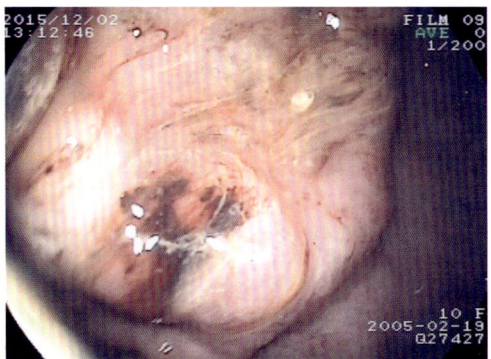 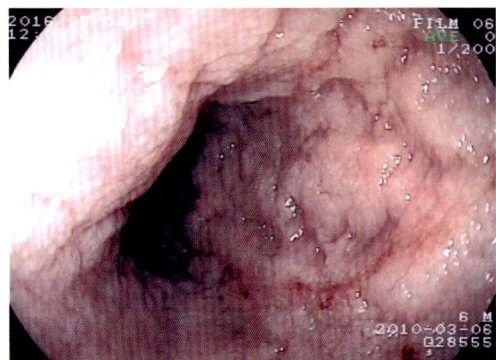

Figure 25. Endoscopic image of a carcinoma in the lesser curvature (incisura angularis) of the stomach.

Figure 26. Endoscopic image of a lymphosarcoma in the small intestine.

Carcinoma is the most common form of stomach cancer in dogs. It is uncommon in cats. The most frequent locations are in the lesser curvature of the gastric corpus (incisura angularis) and the pyloric antrum. In the first case, the tumour tends to present as a large mass with a central ulcer, frequently accompanied by active bleeding (Fig. 25). In the second case, it typically affects the full circumference of the pyloric antrum.

Tumours of the small intestine

Endoscopy is the most useful diagnostic technique for tumours located in the first portions of the digestive tract (gastroduodenoscopy) or in the last portion of the ileum (iliac endoscopy via colonoscopy). An exploratory laparotomy is sometimes needed instead of endoscopy to diagnose tumours located mainly in the jejunum or ileum.

Lymphoma, followed by carcinoma, is the most common tumour of the small intestine in dogs and cats.

Intestinal lymphoma can present as isolated, multiple, or diffuse masses in any part of the small intestine. The diffuse form is the most common form in both dogs and cats. It affects large portions of the small intestine and is seen as irregular erythematous patches often reminiscent of lesions seen in chronic inflammatory bowel disease (Fig. 26).

Carcinoma of the small intestine generally presents as an isolated mass, with a highly variable extension, in any of the portions of the small intestine.

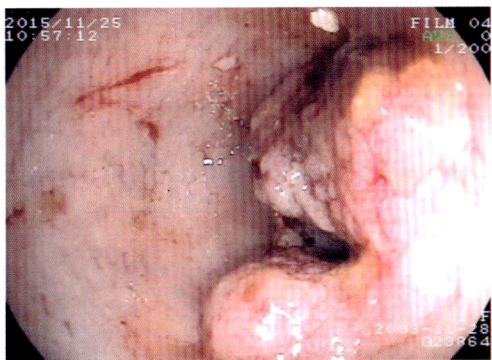

Figure 27. Endoscopic image of a colorectal carcinoma.

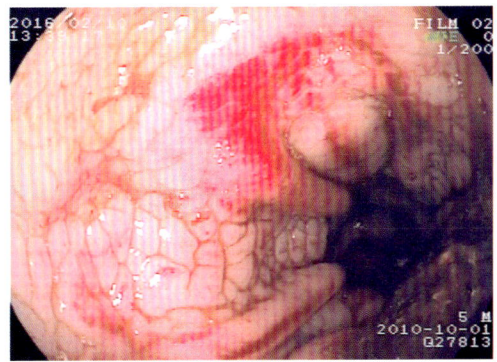

Figure 28. Endoscopic image of a lymphosarcoma in the descending colon.

Tumours of the large intestine

Colonoscopy is the most useful technique for diagnosing tumours of the large intestine. It is used not only to collect specimens for subsequent histopathological study but also to determine the number, size, and location of lesions and the presence of chronic inflammatory bowel disease. Most tumours of the large intestine are located in the rectum or descending colon. Endoscopic biopsy specimens taken from masses in the large intestine must be interpreted with caution in order not to underestimate the severity of disease.

The most common tumours of the large intestine in small animals are polyps (non-neoplastic or inflammatory polyps and true adenomas), carcinomas, and lymphomas. Muscle tumours are very rare.

Inflammatory polyps and **adenomas** tend to have a polypoid appearance and a small implantation base. They are frequently located in the colorectal region and the rectum, close to the anal sphincter.

Carcinomas have a highly varied gross appearance. They can present as a polyp with a wide implantation base or as an extensive mass. On occasions, they can affect the entire circumference of the intestine. Their location also varies greatly, but there is a predilection for the rectum, the colorectal region, and the most distal portion of the descending colon (Fig. 27).

Lymphoma generally presents as multiple masses, although solitary masses have also been described. It is more common in the descending colon and the colorectal region (Fig. 28).

Muscle tumours are rare and tend to occur in the rectal area at the union between the rectum and the anal sphincter. They have also been described in the ascending colon, near the ileocaecal and caecocolic valves.

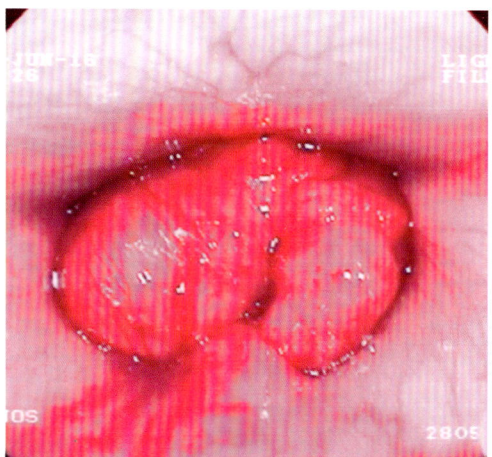
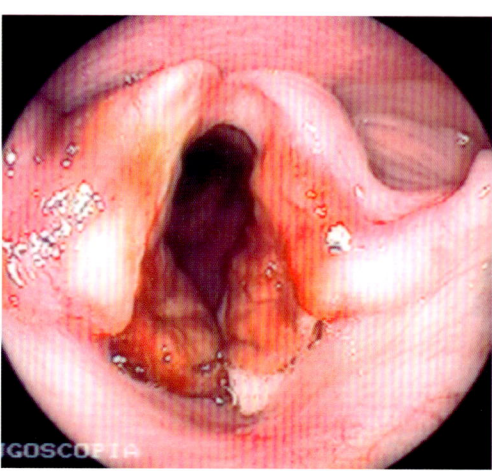

Figure 29. Endoscopic image of a carcinoma in the caudal part of the nostrils.

Figure 30. Endoscopic image of a laryngeal carcinoma.

Airway endoscopy

Airway endoscopy is the most common technique used to diagnose airway tumours. It includes rhinoscopy, laryngoscopy, and tracheobronchoscopy.

Rhinoscopy offers numerous advantages for investigating suspected nasal tumours, as it can pinpoint the location of the tumour, guide the collection of biopsy specimens, and reveal destruction of the nasal septum or turbinates. It also has limitations, however, as in patients with a tumour, it can be difficult to operate in narrow, collapsed, or difficult-to-access areas. Mucus build-up or bleeding can further complicate the procedure. The diagnostic yield of rhinoscopy has been estimated at over 80 %, and is influenced by the experience of the operator and the size of the patient.

Rhinoscopy can be divided into rostral rhinoscopy and caudal rhinoscopy, although the latter is of greater relevance as most nasal tumours are located in the caudal part of the nasal cavity. Carcinomas and sarcomas (Fig. 29), and less so benign tumours, are common. Macroscopically, these tumours are very similar. Laryngeal (Fig. 30) and tracheal (Fig. 31) tumours are relatively uncommon but are easy identifiable by endoscopy. Endoscopic examination of the lower airways is useful for differentiating between tumours and a range of chronic respiratory disorders. Nonetheless, as opposed to humans, lung tumours in dogs and

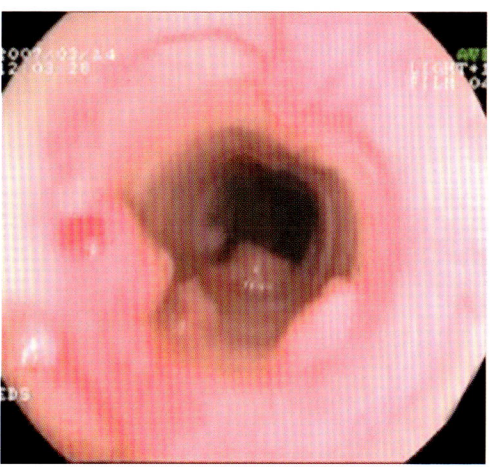 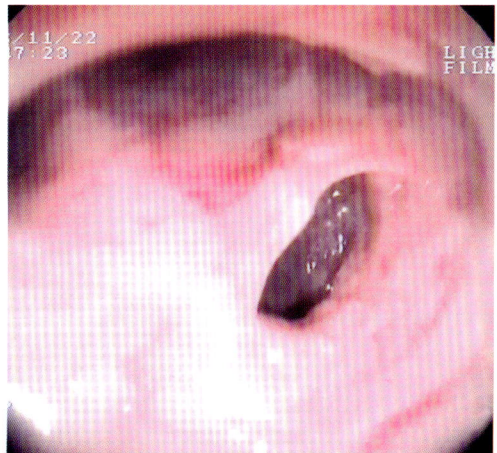

Figure 31. Endoscopic image of a tracheal lymphosarcoma.

Figure 32. Endoscopic image of a pulmonary carcinoma.

cats tend to be associated with minimal or nonexistent mucosal changes, as they usually develop at the periphery. Tumours developing within the ducts are therefore uncommon. For the same reason, endoscopic cytology, which is often used in humans for the diagnosis of endobronchial masses, is less useful in dogs and cats. However, endoscopy can detect airway compression, which appears before the tumour invades the mucosa (Fig. 32). Lesions of the bronchial mucosa, by contrast, are much more common in chronic bronchitis, which tends to present as nodular lesions (caused by fibrosis) that can be confused with tumours.

Endoscopy in other locations

Endoscopy is also useful in the following locations:

Urinary tract. The diagnosis of bladder and urethral tumours is sometimes complicated by the difficulty of collecting samples and the risk of spread by implantation (e.g. in transitional cell carcinoma). Cystoscopy, however, allows clinicians to directly observe a tumour, collect a representative sample, and, where necessary, install a stent.

Musculoskeletal system. Arthroscopy is useful for diagnosing certain tumours, particularly those affecting the joint capsule.

General state of senior patients. Laboratory tests

A full laboratory workup is essential for diagnosing certain haematological malignancies and identifying concomitant disease. The most common concomitant diseases in dogs are periodontal disease, osteoarthritis, heart disease (congestive heart failure, endocarditis), hypothyroidism, diabetes, Cushing's disease, and chronic kidney disease (IRIS stage 1–4), among others. In cats, the most common comorbidities are hypothyroidism, hypertrophic cardiomyopathy, diabetes, chronic kidney disease, and inflammatory bowel disease.

A complete blood count, biochemistry profiles, and a complete urinalysis help to determine the patient's general state of health. This is important not only for guiding treatment strategies but also for establishing a prognosis.

- **Complete blood count and blood smear.** These are essential for evaluating and characterising anaemia, which is a common laboratory finding in patients with cancer. Anaemia can be non-regenerative due to the presence of chronic disease (either the tumour or other conditions), regenerative (due to haemorrhage, such as in HSA), or haemolytic (as occurs in paraneoplastic syndromes). These tests can also rule out other paraneoplastic syndromes, such as erythrocytosis, thrombocytopaenia, and leukocytosis. A blood smear should always be prepared when a complete blood count is performed to check the veracity of data. Detection of morphologically abnormal blood cells can also help to establish a definitive diagnosis (e.g. advanced-stage leukaemia and lymphoma). In other cases, it can help to guide diagnosis. Acanthocytes and schistocytes in a blood smear, for example, are highly suggestive of HSA.
- **Biochemistry.** A complete biochemical profile can help to determine a patient's overall health and rule out concomitant diseases such as chronic kidney disease or liver disease. It can also reveal the presence of paraneoplastic syndromes, such as hypercalcaemia or hypoglycaemia, thus narrowing the differential diagnosis.
- **Electrolytes:** K^+, Na^+, and Cl^-.
- **Complete urinalysis.** A complete urinalysis also provides data on a patient's overall health and kidney function and helps to rule out associated urinary tract infections. On occasions, it can be crucial for establishing a diagnosis (e.g. tumour cells in the sediment of a transitional cell carcinoma or severe proteinuria in MM).

Coagulation tests are essential diagnostic tools in conditions such as HSA and inflammatory carcinoma. Hormones should be measured if an endocrine-related disorder is suspected or if the patient has thyroid cancer (measurement of T_4 and THS before and after surgical excision of the tumour). Finally, in patients with suspected insulinoma, blood insulin levels should be measured as part of the diagnostic workup during an episode of hypoglycaemia with a blood glucose level <70 mg/dl.

Clinical staging: TNM staging system

Clinical stage refers to the extent of a tumour at a given moment. It is essential for deciding on the best treatment strategy and establishing a prognosis. To stage a tumour it is necessary to know the size of the tumour (T), the degree to which regional lymph nodes are involved (N), and presence of distant metastasis (M). As each tumour has a different biological behaviour, different clinical staging systems are used depending on the type of tumour. The most common system used in veterinary oncology is the World Health Organization's TNM Classification of Tumours in Domestic Animals, edited by Owen (1980) (Table 3). All the diagnostic procedures described in this chapter, combined with investigation of systemic involvement, help to establish clinical stage.

Table 3. **World Health Organization TNM Classification of Tumours in Domestic Animals**

Code	Significance
T: primary tumour	
T0	No evidence of tumour
Tis	Carcinoma in situ
T1	Primary tumour <3 cm
T2	Tumour 3–5 cm
T3	Tumour >5 cm
T4	Invasion of adjacent structures
N: regional lymph nodes	
N0	No evidence of regional lymph node involvement
N1	Movable ipsilateral nodes
N2	Movable contralateral nodes
N3	Fixed nodes
M: metastasis	
M0	No distant metastasis
M1	Distant metastasis detected

4

Diagnostic interpretation, choice of treatment, and prognosis

Cytology

A cytology sample is considered adequate when it has a high content of tissue cells. The following points should be borne in mind when establishing a cytological diagnosis:
- A negative result can **never** rule out a diagnosis of cancer. Tumour samples may contain insufficient cells with which to establish a diagnosis. This can occur with tumours that do not exfoliate readily or with samples contaminated with blood during collection. Tumours are heterogeneous masses that may contain both inflammatory and necrotic components. Detection of inflammatory cells and/or microorganisms thus does not rule out cancer.
- There is a very fine line between a benign tumour (or even a well-differentiated malignant tumour) and hyperplastic or normal tissue.
- In inflammatory conditions, tissue cells undergo dysplastic changes that are cytologically indistinguishable from neoplastic changes. This is more common in cavity effusions or certain tissues (e.g. bladder tissue in urine samples).
- Observation of tissue cells with malignant features is strongly suggestive of malignancy.
- In some tissues, malignant cells do not always show dramatic changes (e.g. perianal gland tumour cells), and as such, the absence of sufficient criteria for malignancy does not necessarily exclude a diagnosis of cancer.
- Poorly differentiated tumours often lack characteristic cell features that indicate their origin.
- When evaluating cytology samples from internal organs, it is essential to be familiar with the characteristics of the normal cell population to avoid confusion with neoplastic changes.

Cytological assessment of cell lineage

There are three basic tissue types in tumours (Fig. 1): epithelial, mesenchymal, (Fig. 2), and round-cell (Fig. 3) (Table 1).

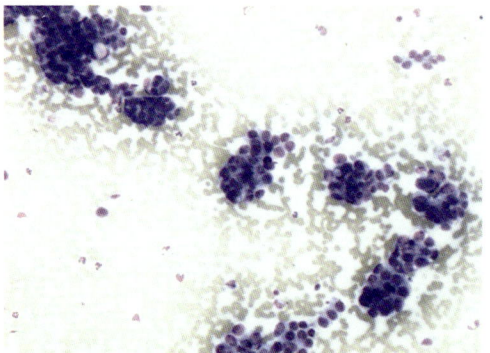

Figure 1. Cytology of an epithelial tumour showing clusters of cell (May–Grünwald–Giemsa, ×10 objective).

Diagnostic interpretation, choice of treatment, and prognosis

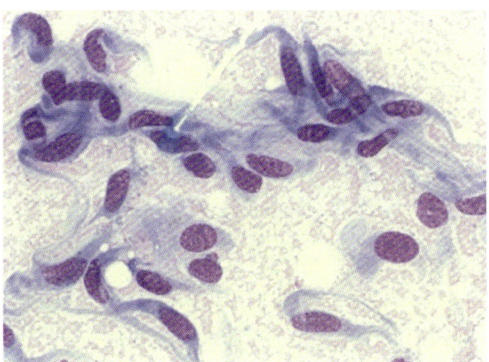

Figure 2. Cytology of a mesenchymal tumour showing the typical spindle-like cell morphology (May–Grünwald–Giemsa, ×40 objective).

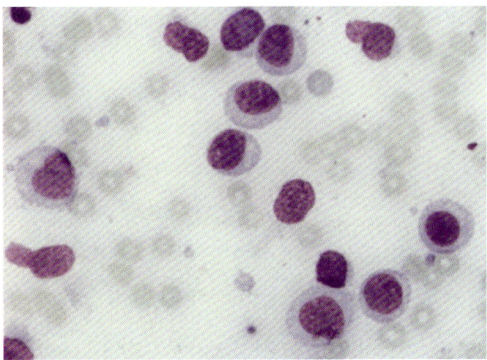

Figure 3. Cytology of a round-cell tumour (histiocytoma) showing the round morphology of the cells (May–Grünwald–Giemsa, ×40 objective).

Table 1. Cytological characteristics of normal tissue according to its origin.

Characteristic	Epithelial tissue	Mesenchymal tissue	Round-cell tissue
Cellularity	High	Low	High
Cell distribution	Groups	Individual	Individual
Size	Large	Medium–small	Medium–small
Shape	Round–polyhedral	Spindle–oval	Round
Cytoplasmic borders	Well-defined	Poorly defined	Well-defined
Nucleus	Round, eccentric	Round–oval	Round, central

Assessment of cytological criteria for malignancy

There are three groups of criteria for determining malignancy: cellular criteria, nuclear criteria, and cytoplasmic criteria.

General cytological criteria
- Increased cellularity (valid only for mesenchymal tumours).
- Voluminous, disorganised groups of cells (epithelial tumours).
- Cellular pleomorphism: cells of different shapes and sizes, except in round-cell tumours, which have a monomorphic cell population.
- Mitosis. A high mitotic rate generally indicates malignancy, although it must always be considered within the context of the tumour being evaluated. Abnormal or atypical mitoses are a much stronger indicator of malignancy (Fig. 4).

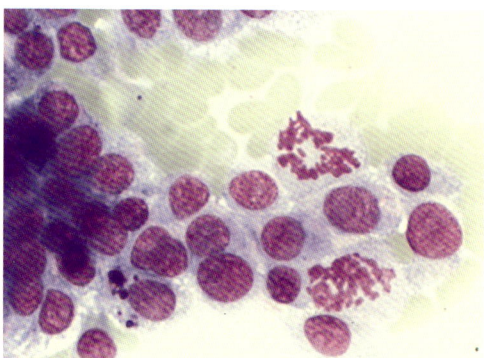

Figure 4. Atypical mitosis in a malignant epithelial tumour (May–Grünwald–Giemsa, ×40 objective).

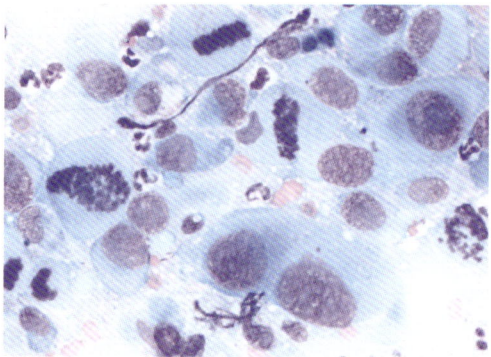

Figure 5. Malignant tumour showing numerous nuclear criteria of malignancy (May–Grünwald–Giemsa, ×100 objective).

Nuclear criteria. These are the most important criteria for establishing degree of malignancy (Fig. 5).
- Increased nuclear size.
- Increased nucleus:cytoplasm ratio.
- Anisokaryosis.
- Increased, irregular chromatin clumping.
- Increased number and size of nucleoli.
- Multiple and/or irregular nuclei, with images of nuclear moulding.

Cytoplasmic criteria. Cytoplasmic changes are the result of an increased or abnormal synthesis of cytoplasm or a lack of differentiation.
- Marked cytoplasmic basophilia.
- Vacuolisation.
- Images of false phagocytes.
- Loss of specific cytoplasmic granules.

Cytoplasmic changes are always considered to be complementary to nuclear changes, which are more useful for identifying cell lineage.

Generally speaking, the detection of ≥3 nuclear criteria or ≥4 general criteria indicates that a tumour is malignant. At least 5 nuclear criteria for malignancy are required to diagnose a mesothelioma, as both normal and reactive mesothelial cells in cavity effusion samples have very evident dysplastic features.

Cytological characteristics of main tumours
Epithelial tumours

Epithelial tumours are classified as glandular or nonglandular depending on the respective presence or absence of cytoplasmic vacuoles. Glandular tumours are characterised by either very prominent vacuoles (e.g. macrovacuoles or signet-ring cells in sebaceous gland tumours [Fig. 6], exocrine pancreatic tumours, and salivary gland tumours) or microvacuoles that gives the cytoplasm a "moth-eaten" appearance (e.g. in perianal gland tumours [Fig. 7] or prostate samples). Although liver tissue is not glandular, its cells also have a highly characteristic moth-eaten appearance. Nonglandular tumours (basal cell or hair follicle tumours) do not have vacuoles (Fig. 8).

Neuroendocrine tissue is an epithelial tissue that displays similar characteristics regardless of its origin (thyroid gland, hepatic neuroendocrine tumours, adrenal gland, etc.). Cells have a moderate clear or lightly basophilic cytoplasm and large groups of cells with indistinguishable borders. Cytological features thus tend to include naked nuclei against a basophilic background where only some cells have a distinguishable cytoplasmic border (Fig. 9).

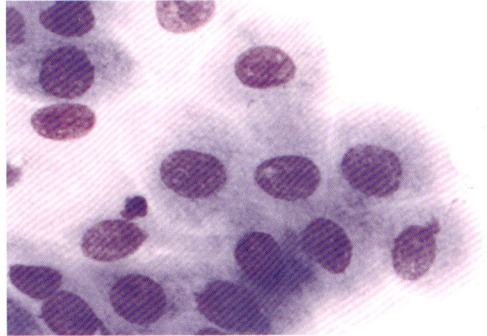

Figure 7. Perianal gland tumour with microvacuolated or "moth-eaten" cytoplasm (May–Grünwald–Giemsa, ×100 objective).

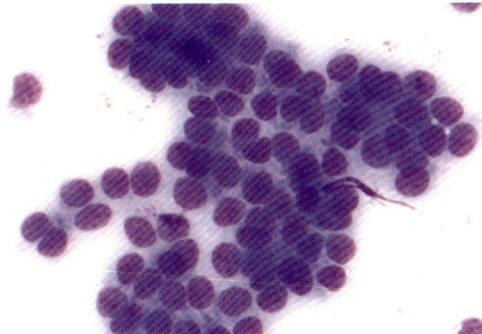

Figure 8. Nonglandular epithelial tumour (basal cell tumour) (May–Grünwald–Giemsa, ×40 objective).

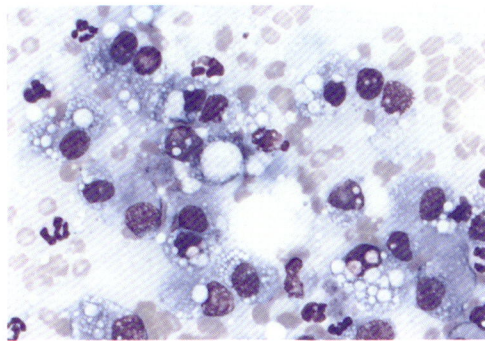

Figure 6. Glandular epithelial tumour with characteristic cytoplasmic macrovacuoles (May–Grünwald–Giemsa, ×40 objective).

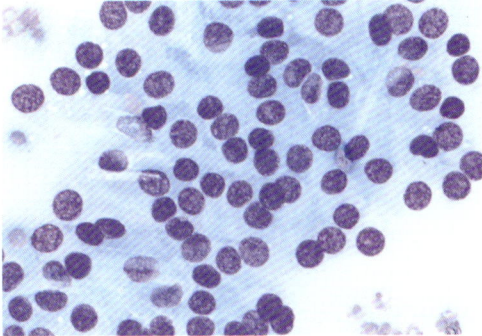

Figure 9. Neuroendocrine tumour with indistinguishable cell borders (May–Grünwald–Giemsa, ×40 objective).

Mesenchymal tumours

Benign mesenchymal tumours (fibroma, leiomyoma) are very difficult to diagnose cytologically as they tend to exfoliate poorly. Their malignant counterparts, by contrast, show abundant cells with differing degrees of atypia. The main objective of diagnostic cytology in mesenchymal tumours is to differentiate between low- and high-grade sarcomas.

Cells in low-grade **sarcomas** (Fig. 10) typically exfoliate in high numbers and may form "pseudogroups". The cells show atypia (but with <3 nuclear criteria of malignancy) and occasional mitoses. High-grade sarcomas (Fig. 11), regardless of their origin, are highly anaplastic and show clear general criteria for malignancy and numerous atypical mitoses.

Approximately 50 % of injection-site sarcomas (ISSs) can be diagnosed cytologically. The features in this case are similar to those of a high-grade sarcoma with numerous giant multinucleated cells.

Osteosarcoma (OSA) has different characteristics to other sarcomas (Fig. 12). Neoplastic cells (osteoblasts) are small to medium in size, have a round–oval shape, a strongly basophilic cytoplasm, and a largely eccentric nucleus. They are thus similar to plasma cells. Osteoclasts (multinucleated cells) distributed within a bright pink osteoid/chondroid matrix are very common.

Round-cell tumours

Well-differentiated round-cell tumours are in general the easiest tumours to identify, as they have clear cell characteristics. Diagnosis, however, can be very complicated in undifferentiated tumours.

Histiocytoma cells have a wide cytoplasm and, on occasions, small vacuoles. The nuclei

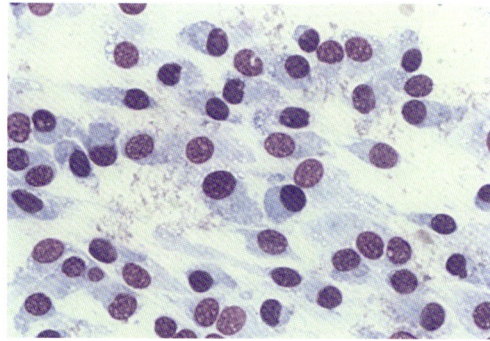

Figure 10. Low-grade sarcoma with little evidence of malignancy (May–Grünwald–Giemsa, ×40 objective).

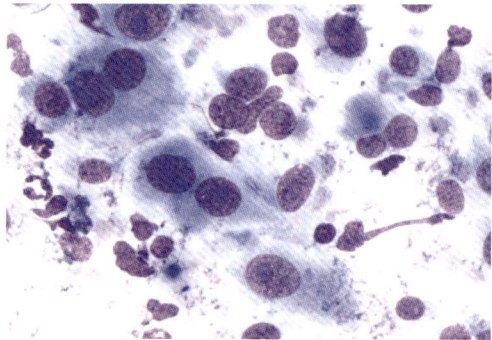

Figure 11. High-grade sarcoma with very evident atypia (May–Grünwald–Giemsa, ×100 objective).

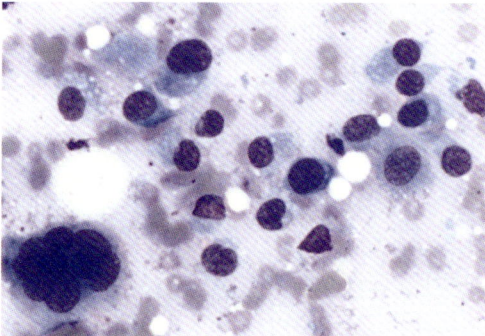

Figure 12. Osteosarcoma with round–oval osteoblasts and an osteoclast (multinucleated cell) (May–Grünwald–Giemsa, ×40 objective).

are often kidney-shaped. **Histiocytic sarcoma** cells show clear criteria for malignancy (Fig. 13).

Mast cell tumour (MCT) cells have metachromatic cytoplasmic granules (Figs. 14

Diagnostic interpretation, choice of treatment, and prognosis

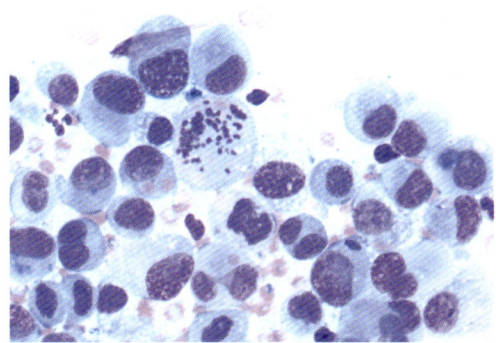

Figure 13. Histiocytic sarcoma. Note the kidney-shaped nuclei with evident atypia and atypical central mitosis (May-Grünwald-Giemsa, ×40 objective).

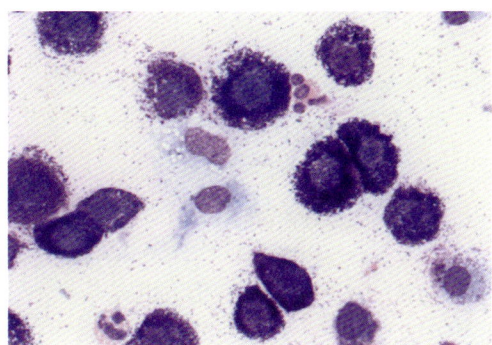

Figure 14. Well-differentiated mast cell tumour (May-Grünwald-Giemsa, ×40 objective).

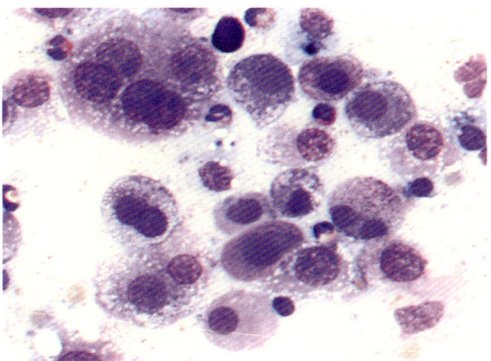

Figure 15. An estimated undifferentiated mast cell tumour (May-Grünwald-Giemsa, ×40 objective).

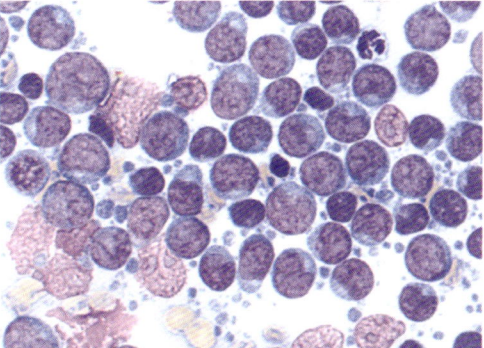

Figure 16. Cytology of a lymph node. Note the monomorphic features and predominance of lymphoblasts, characteristic of lymphoma (May-Grünwald-Giemsa, ×100 objective).

and 15). Cytological grade (well differentiated or undifferentiated) can be estimated based on the number or size of granules and the presence or absence of atypia. Most MCTs have an eosinophilic infiltrate and very active mesenchymal cells.

Transmissible venereal tumour (TVT) cells have a wide cytoplasm with a variable number of small clear vacuoles of varying shapes.

Lymphosarcomas (LSAs) contain numerous lymphoblasts, which are cells of varying sizes (depending on the stage of maturation) that have a large round nucleus and an intensely basophilic cytoplasm with a characteristic half-moon appearance. Most LSAs involve the lymph nodes, and the associated cytological diagnostic yield is estimated at 90 % (Fig. 16). The pleomorphic image of a normal or reactive lymph node with a predominance of mature lymphocytes is replaced by a monomorphic population of lymphoblasts, which account for >50 % of the lymphoid population. In low-grade LSAs, it is difficult to differentiate between tumour cells and normal cells.

Lymphoblasts in samples taken from the skin, effusions, or internal organs (spleen, liver, kidneys) are strongly diagnostic for LSA.

Melanomas

Melanomas do not have a characteristic cell type, as they can contain epithelial, mesenchymal, or round cells, and sometimes even a combination of these in the same area (Fig. 17). Detection of melanin granules can aid diagnosis except in the case of amelanotic melanomas.

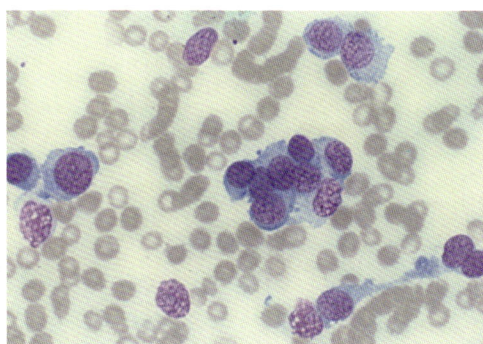

Figure 17. Cytology of an amelanotic melanoma. Note the cells with features showing different lineages (May-Grünwald-Giemsa, ×40 objective).

Biopsy

Histopathological examination is of diagnostic aid and can help to identify and determine the extent of disease, tumour grade, and the relationship between the tumour and other tissues. This information, together with clinical stage, is essential for establishing a prognosis and deciding on the best course of treatment.

It is important to understand the following terms that typically appear in biopsy reports:
- Dysplasia: non-tumoural tissue changes.
- Hyperplasia: increased cell numbers.
- Metaplasia: transformation of one cell type to another.
- Anaplasia: loss of morphological characteristics of original tissue cells.
- Pleomorphism: variability in cell shape and size.
- Scirrhous response: proliferation of fibroblasts in certain malignant tumours.
- In situ: malignant tumour that has not penetrated the basal membrane.
- Adenoma/papilloma/epithelioma: benign tumour of epithelial origin.
- Carcinoma: malignant tumour of epithelial origin.
- Adenocarcinoma: malignant tumour of epithelial origin that arises in the gland cells.
- Sarcoma: malignant tumour of mesenchymal origin.

What is tumour grade?

Tumour grade refers to a tumour's growth rate and ability to spread. Well-differentiated tumours contain cells that are similar to those found in normal tissue and are characterised by relatively slow growth and a poor ability to spread. Poorly differentiated or undifferentiated tumours, by contrast, grow fast and are able to invade adjacent tissues and/or spread to other sites.

Different systems exist for calculating tumour grade, but they all share a numerical rating system that grades the tumour on a scale of 1–3 or 1–4. Grade 1 describes tumours with similar cells and structure to those of the original tissue. These characteristics are gradually lost with increasing tumour grade. Generally speaking:

- G0: grade cannot be assessed (undetermined grade).
- G1: well-differentiated (low-grade) (Fig. 18).
- G2: moderately differentiated (intermediate-grade).
- G3: poorly differentiated (high-grade) (Fig. 19).
- G4: undifferentiated (high-grade).

Some tumours have a specific grading system (e.g. breast cancer, which involves assessment of tubule formation).

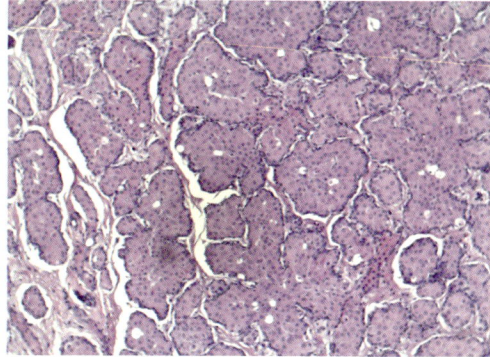

Figure 18. Histopathological image (H&E) of a hepatoid adenoma.

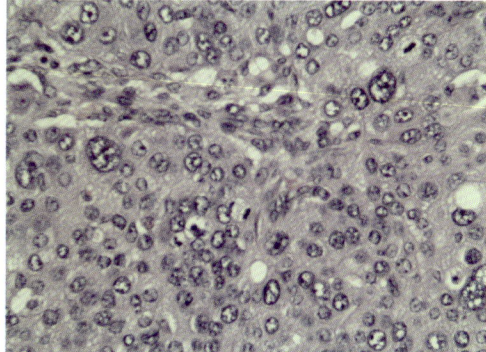

Figure 19. Histopathological image (H&E) of a high-grade transitional cell carcinoma of the bladder.

Tumour margins

Histopathological examination is also used by pathologists to determine whether or not a tumour has been completely excised. This is done by analysing the deep and lateral margins and requires close communication between the pathologist and the surgeon.

As a general rule, margins extending <1 mm from the cut margin (healthy tissue) are considered to be insufficient (narrow margins), while those located between 1 and 3 mm are considered to be safe (clear margins). This rule, however, is not applicable to all tumours (Figs. 20–22).

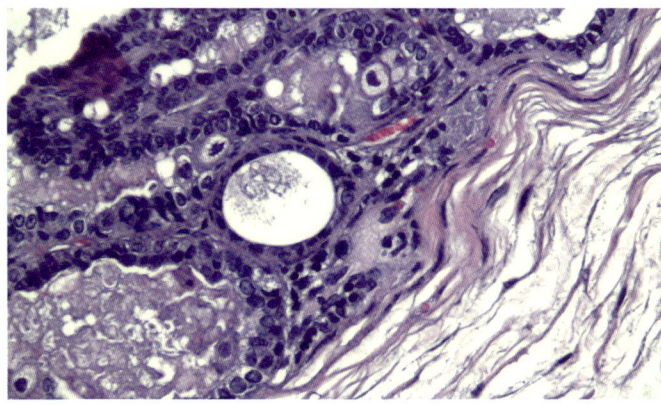

Figure 20. Biopsy section (H&E) of a mammary tumour showing clean borders (×40 objective).

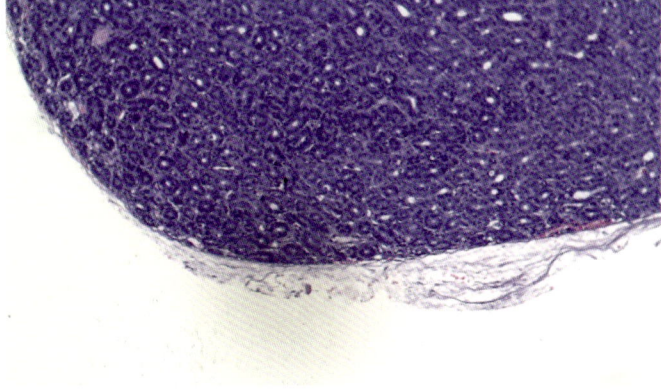

Figure 21. Biopsy section (H&E) of a mammary tumour showing narrow borders (×10 objective).

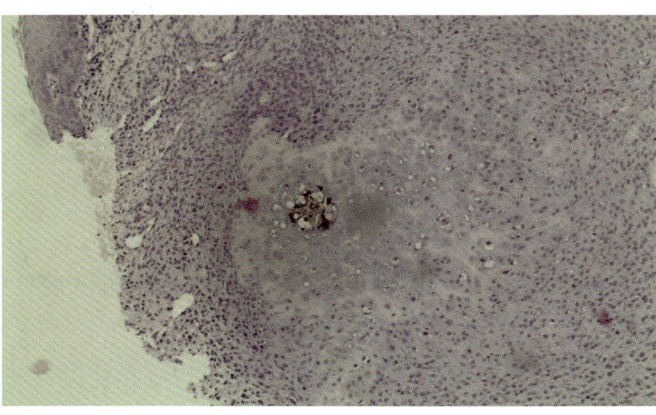

Figure 22. Biopsy section (H&E) of an oral chondrosarcoma showing dirty borders (×10 objective).

Special stains

Routine staining with haematoxylin–eosin (H&E) cannot always identify the origin of the tissue. This is the case, for example, with highly aggressive tumours (anaplastic tumours), which require the use of special stains (other than H&E or immunohistochemical [IHC] stains) to identify the origin of the tissue and even the proliferative ability of the tumour. Examples of these stains are:

- Toluidine blue: used to identify granules in mast cells that cannot be identified with H&E.
- Masson trichrome: used to identify collagen in mesenchymal tumours arising in muscle tissue (leiomyoma, leiomyosarcoma, rhabdomyoma, rhabdomyosarcoma) or connective tissue (fibrosarcoma [FSA]).
- IHC stains: stains containing antibodies directed against specific molecules.
  - Vimentin: used to identify intermediate filaments of mesenchymal origin.
  - Cytokeratin: used to identify tumours of epithelial origin.
  - Desmin: used to identify tumours of muscle origin.
  - Factor VII antigens: used to identify tumours of endothelial origin.
  - S-100 protein: used to identify melanomas.
  - Ki-67: used to determine cell proliferation rate (Fig 23).
  - T-cell and B-cell markers (CD3 and CD79a, respectively).
  - CD117: used to identify C-KIT protein (MCT).

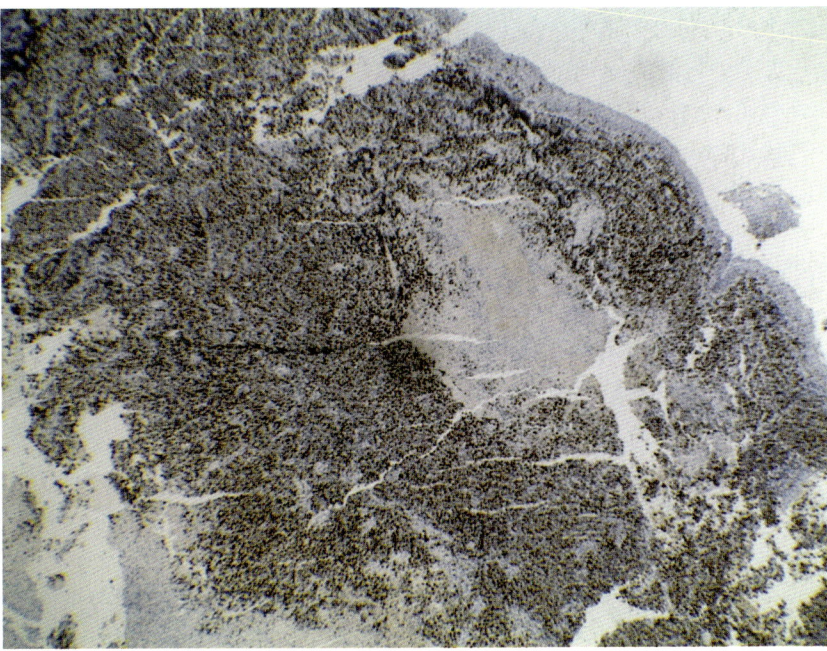

Figure 23. Ki-67 staining of a high-grade lymphosarcoma.

Biological behaviour of tumours according to tissue of origin

Epithelial tumours

Epithelial tumours arise in cutaneous epithelial tissue, in organ- or structure-lining tissue, or in gland tissue. Most tumours of this type develop on the skin surface (follicular tumours, sebaceous tumours, squamous cell carcinoma [SCC]) or in the dermis (mammary gland, perianal tumours), and are therefore readily noticed by owners. Internal tumours that run an asymptomatic, insidious course are often not detected until they are already at an advanced stage. The most common epithelial neoplasms are as follows:

The most common epithelial tumours are (Fig. 24):
- Adenoma/sebaceous gland carcinoma.
- Follicular tumours.
- Squamous cell carcinoma.
- Bronchoalveolar carcinoma.
- Mammary tumours of epithelial origin.
- Adenoma/carcinoma of the liver, colon, stomach, intestine, kidney, bladder, pancreas, prostate, adrenal glands, or anal sac.
- Neuroendocrine tumours of the uterus, ovaries, prostate, or testicles.

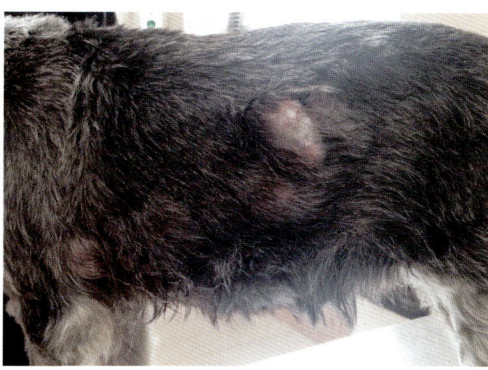

Figure 24. Nonspayed 12-year-old Schnauzer with multiple skin lesions cytologically consistent with carcinoma.

The above carcinomas tend to metastasise with a preference for the lungs, liver, bladder, brain, and to a lesser extent, the skin and bone. Metastatic lesions tend to present as slow-growing nodules. The clinical signs are directly related to the location of the tumour and sometimes to the presence of paraneoplastic syndromes (e.g. hypercalcaemia secondary to anal sac carcinoma).

Mesenchymal tumours

Mesenchymal tumours are derived from mesenchymal, endothelial, and muscle tissue (smooth and skeletal). Although depending on their location and biological behaviour, mesenchymal tumours can be benign or malignant, most of them run a malignant course and are characterised by invasive growth and poorly circumscribed margins. Surgical excision with wide margins is therefore often not possible and recurrence rates are high. Computed tomography (CT) is the technique of choice for establishing clinical stage and planning surgery. The likelihood of distant metastasis depends on tumour grade. Because response to chemotherapy is poor in mesenchymal tumours, patients in whom surgery is unsuccessful are generally administered radiation therapy.

The main types of mesenchymal tumours are:
- **Soft-tissue sarcoma.** Soft-tissue sarcoma (STS) accounts for 15 % of all cutaneous and subcutaneous tumours in dogs (Fig. 25). Examples are FSA, nerve sheath tumours, haemangiopericytoma, myxosarcoma, liposarcoma, synovial cell sarcoma, leiomyosarcoma, and rhabdomyosarcoma. Cytological diagnosis is often not possible due to the associated inflammatory component (see section *"Biological behaviour of tumour according to location"*).
- **Injection-site sarcoma.** Feline injection-site sarcoma (ISS) is associated with the injection of irritant substances in cats (Fig. 26). It is characterised by fast-growing masses that appear weeks or months after injection. Approximately 25 % of cats may have lung metastasis at the time of diagnosis. Recurrence is high (90 % at 6–12 months of surgery) and there is invasion and destruction of peripheral tissues.
- **Bone sarcomas** (Fig. 27). Osteosarcoma (OSA) is the most common primary form of bone sarcoma, although other forms, including chondrosarcomas, are possible. OSA is an aggressive tumour with high metastatic potential in dogs (90 % have micrometastases at diagnosis). In cats, surgery tends to be curative. Although OSA can affect dogs of any age, large and giant breeds are at greater risk.

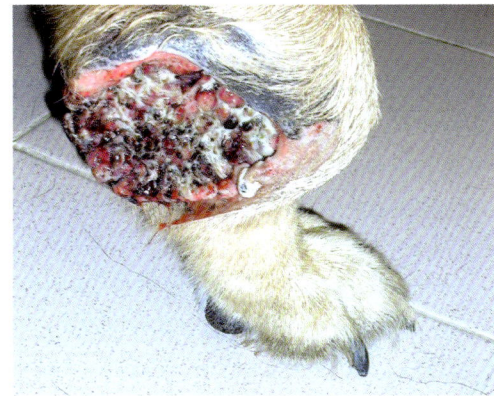

Figure 25. Ulcerated soft-tissue sarcoma on the right forelimb of a German Shepherd.

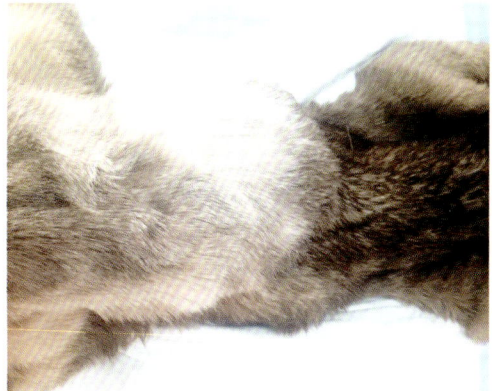

Figure 26. Interscapular injection-site sarcoma in a 14-year-old male cat. Note the cachexia.

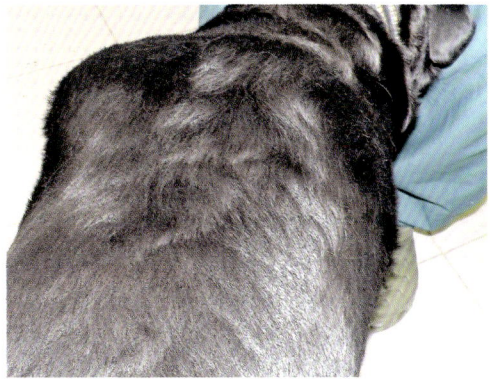

Figure 27. Mass (with cytological findings consistent with osteosarcoma) on the scapula of the left forelimb of a female Rottweiler.

Haematopoietic tumours

Haematopoietic tumours originate in lymphoid organs (where they are known as LSAs or lymphomas) or, less frequently, in bone marrow (leukaemia).

Lymphosarcoma is the most common haematopoietic tumour in **dogs** and it tends to affect elderly individuals (aged 6–12 years). It can affect any organ and is classified according to anatomical location or lymphocyte population. In the first case, it is classified as multicentric, which accounts for 80 % of all LSAs in dogs (Fig. 8), alimentary, mediastinal, or extranodal (skin, kidneys, nervous system, eyes). In the second case, a distinction is made between B-cell lymphoma and T-cell lymphoma (which normally has a worse prognosis). Eventually, LSA spreads to other organs (liver, spleen, bone marrow, lymph nodes) (Table 2). Finally, indolent LSA is a variant that is characterised by a slow, insidious course.

If the cytology or biopsy results are inconclusive, more advanced diagnostic techniques such as flow cytometry or PCR for antigen receptor rearrangements (PARR) are necessary (see Chapter 3).

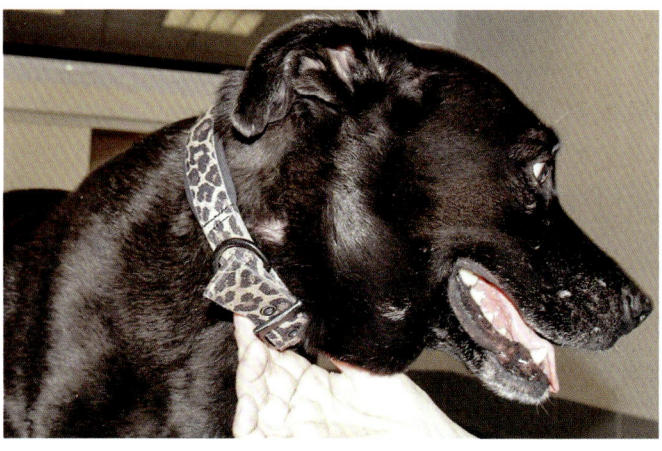

Figure 28. Generalised lymphadenopathy in a mixed-breed female with cytological findings consistent with multicentric lymphosarcoma.

Lymphosarcoma is one of the most common **feline** tumours and affects an estimated 200 of every 100,000 cats at risk. The most common variants in these animals are mediastinal, alimentary, and extranodal (nasal, renal, nervous system, ocular, and cutaneous). It occurs in two age groups of cats that are distinguishable by the presence or absence of feline leukaemia virus (FeVL):
- young cats (around 2 years of age), which are normally FeVL-positive and develop mediastinal LSA;
- and older cats (8–12 years of age), which are normally FeVL-negative and develop alimentary LSA.

Feline immunodeficiency virus has also been linked to the development of LSA.

Table 2. Clinical stages for multicentric canine lymphosarcoma according to the WHO.

Clinical stage	Characteristics	
I	Involvement of a single lymph node or lymphoid tissue in a single organ (e.g. spleen)	
II	Regional involvement of multiple lymph nodes on one side of the diaphragm	
III	Generalised lymph node enlargement (of all palpable lymph nodes)	
IV	Involvement of the liver and/or spleen	
V	Bone marrow involvement[1]	
For all stages:	Substage a	Without systemic signs of disease
	Substage b	With systemic signs of disease

[1] Stage V can imply substage b. Typical signs of bone marrow invasion are the characteristic signs of myelophthisis, with suppression of red blood cells and platelets (as a direct consequence of the tumour). Secondary hypercalcaemia is also a possibility.

Alimentary LSA is generally diffuse and can sometimes be difficult to distinguish from lymphocytic–plasmacytic inflammatory bowel disease. Most cases of LSA involving the intestinal mucosa are small-cell LSAs, while most transmural cases are large-cell LSAs. Feline large granular lymphocyte LSA is a particularly aggressive type of alimentary LSA and can involve T cells or natural killer cells.

Other origins

Nervous system tumours are difficult to diagnose and treat (see Chapter 3).

The main tumours caused by **histiocytic disorders** are:
- Reactive cutaneous histiocytosis, which is a benign reactive proliferation with a fibroblastic component.
- Canine cutaneous histiocytoma, which arises in Langerhans cells. This condition is normally self-limiting but there are persistent and recurrent variants. Langerhans cell histiocytosis can progress to systemic disease.
- Histiocytic sarcoma, previously known as malignant histiocytosis, has a localised and a disseminated form. The latter can affect the spleen, lymph nodes, visceral organs, eyes, central nervous system (CNS), and skin. Rottweilers, Bernese Mountain Dogs, Golden Retrievers, Labrador Retrievers, and miniature Schnauzers have a greater disposition to histiocytic sarcoma. Cats can also develop this tumour, but the risk is lower. The tumour invades and destroys different tissues. The disseminated form is fatal.
- Reactive histiocytosis, which is a non-neoplastic disorder characterised by a reactive perivascular proliferation of antigen-presenting dendritic cells. Cutaneous and systemic forms exist, although they both arise in the skin.

Biological behaviour of tumours according to location

Cutaneous and subcutaneous tumours

Cutaneous and subcutaneous tumours account for approximately 33 % of tumours in dogs and 25 % of those in cats. Approximately 70–80 % of these tumours are benign in dogs compared with 35–50 % in cats.

They can be classified according to:
- Tumour grade: differentiated, moderately differentiated, or undifferentiated
- TMN clinical stage (Tables 3 and 4): LSA and MCTs have separate classification systems.

Clinical presentation varies according to tumour type, anatomical location, time since onset, disease course, bacterial infection, and self-mutilation. Cytology is necessary, but biopsy is essential for establishing a definitive diagnosis. Enlarged regional lymph nodes must be investigated by fine-needle puncture to rule out metastasis.

Prognosis can be influenced by anatomical location (e.g. cutaneous or subungual SCC), species, or even breed.

Table 3. TNM classification of cutaneous tumours in domestic animals (excluding lymphosarcoma and mast cell tumours) (Owen, 1980).

	T system (Primary tumour)[1]		N system (Regional lymph nodes)		M system (Metastasis)
Tis	Carcinoma in situ	N0	No evidence of regional lymph node involvement	M0	No evidence of distant metastasis
T1	<2 cm, noninvasive	N1	Movable ipsilateral nodes	M1	Distant metastasis detected
T2	2–5 cm or minimal invasion	N2	Movable contralateral or bilateral lymph nodes		
T3	>5 cm or with subcutaneous invasion	N3	Fixed nodes		
T4	Tumour invading other structures				

[1] T is defined by the largest tumour when >1 tumour is present.

Table 4. Clinical stages of tumours according to the TNM system.

Clinical stage	TNM classification
I	T1, N0, M0
II	T2, N0, M0
III	T3, N0, M0
IV	TX, N1-2-3, M0
V	TX, NX, M1

NON-NEOPLASTIC LESIONS

Non-neoplastic lesions must be contemplated in the differential diagnosis of cutaneous and subcutaneous tumours. These include:

Hamartomas. Benign nodules caused by the excessive, disorganised growth of mature cells. They present as solitary, well-defined nodules surrounded by skin. They can be congenital (nevi) or acquired (Fig. 29).

Actinic keratosis. There is some debate on whether actinic keratosis should actually be called actinic carcinoma in situ as it has similar genetic and molecular alterations to SCC, affects similar areas (Fig. 30), has a similar aetiology, and sometimes even progresses to SCC.

Cysts.
- Follicular: derived from the outer root sheath of hair follicles; they present as solitary pigmented alopecic dermal or subcutaneous nodules.
- Dermoid: cutaneous structures resembling dermal or subcutaneous masses (Fig. 31).
- Sebaceous: skin-covered sac-like structures filled with sebum.
- Apocrine: well-defined bulbous nodules that contain a bluish or reddish fluid and affect the head, neck, limbs, and dorsal region of dogs. In cats they are typically found in the external ear canal.

Nodular sebaceous hyperplasia (senile sebaceous hyperplasia). Accounts for 25 % of non-neoplastic cutaneous nodules in dogs and 11 % of those in cats. It is caused by an accumulation of nearly mature sebaceous glands in the head, neck, or ears, and is particularly common in Poodles and Cocker Spaniels. In cats, nodular sebaceous hyperplasia tends to present as a solitary lesion on the head and shows a predilection for males.

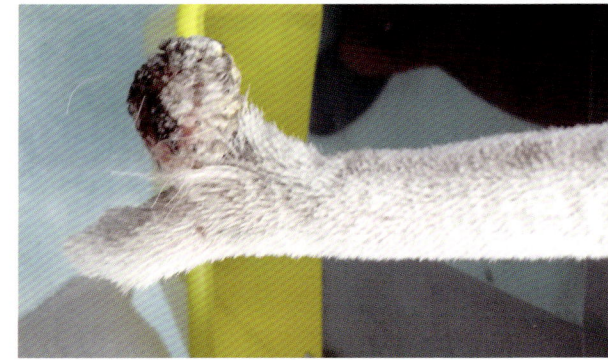

Figure 29. Fibroadnexal hamartoma on the tail of a cat.

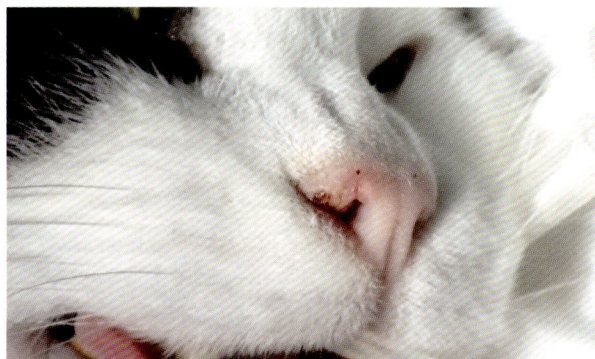

Figure 30. Actinic keratosis on the nose of a cat.

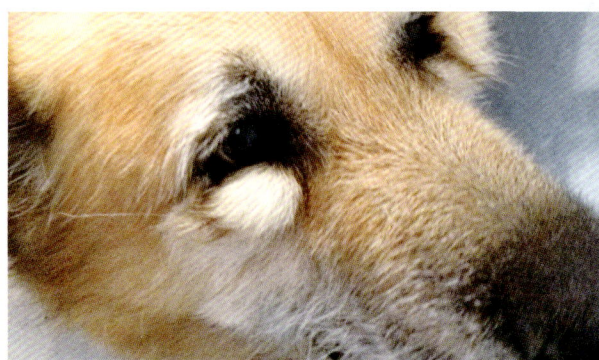

Figure 31. Dermoid cysts of the eyelids.

Acrochordon (fibromatous plaque or fibroepithelial polyp). Solitary or multiple nodules on the trunk that are particularly common at pressure points. They have a polypoid or filiform appearance.

Epithelial tumours of the epidermis

- **Squamous papilloma.** Pedunculated mass on the head, limbs, or genitals. It appears as a solitary lesion in elderly animals and shows a predilection for Cocker Spaniels (Fig. 32).
- **Viral papilloma.** More common in dogs up to 3 years of age. It is contagious and is caused by a DNA virus (incubation period of 1 month). It has a slightly fissured appearance and coliform shape that is round at one end and pedunculated towards the other (Fig. 33). Viral papilloma normally affects the mucosa and generally resolves spontaneously within approximately 3 months (except in immunodepressed patients). Surgery and cryosurgery are the first-line choices when treatment is required, although retinoids may also be considered.
- **Cutaneous squamous cell tumour.** This is the most common malignant tumour in cats and the second most common one in dogs. The mean age of onset is 10 years in cats and 11 in dogs. The main predisposing factor is exposure to ultraviolet radiation and risk factors are a white coat in cats (13-fold increased risk) and a white or scant coat in the ventral region of dogs. Golden and Labrador Retrievers have a greater risk of SCC of the nasal plane. SCC of the nail bed is more common in large dogs with a dark coat and it can spread to regional lymph nodes. In cats, SCC occurs on the head, ears, nose, or eyelids. Approximately 50 % of cats have regional metastasis and distant metastasis involving the nose. Multiple forms are seen in both dogs and cats (Fig. 34) and can vary greatly in appearance, with tumours taking the form of erythematous, crusted, or ulcerated lesions. When it involves the nail bed, SCC presents as an inflammatory lesion with digital deformation (Fig. 35) and osteolysis of the phalanx (Fig. 36). Nail bed SCC accounts for 47 % of all nail bed tumours. The vast majority of lesions are solitary, with multiple lesions seen in just 3 % of cases. Mean age of presentation is 10 years.
  - Prognosis is influenced by tumour grade and adequate surgical excision with wide margins. New lesions frequently occur in the same area if preventive measures are not taken. Nasal and subungual SCC have a worse prognosis.
  - Treatment. Radiation therapy, cryosurgery, intralesional chemotherapy, and photodynamic therapy may be indicated in the early stages of SCC of the nasal plane, although they do not guarantee clear margins. Amputation of the affected digit is necessary in subungual SCC. Recurrence rather than distant metastasis is the most common reason for treatment failure in SCC.

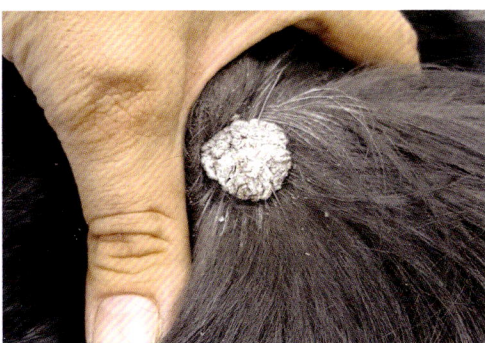

Figure 32. Squamous cell papilloma.

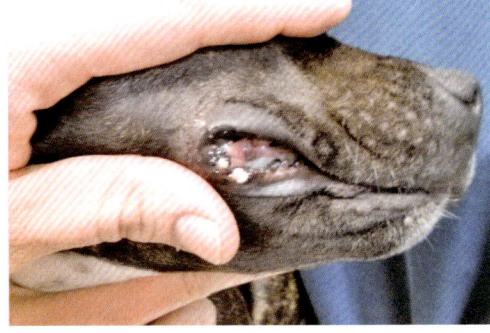

Figure 33. Several viral papillomas on the oral mucosa of a dog.

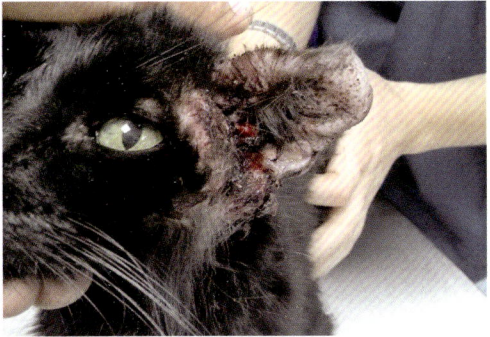

Figure 34. Squamous cell carcinoma on the ear of a cat.

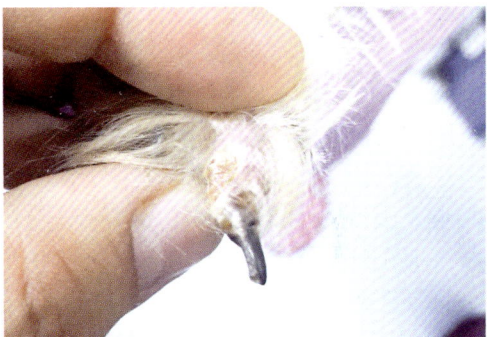

Figure 35. Subungual squamous cell carcinoma.

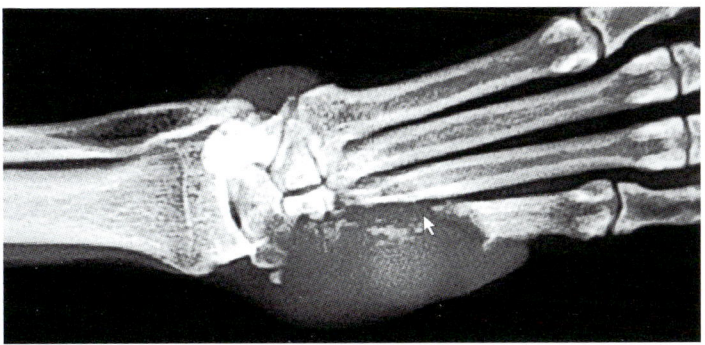

Figure 36. Extensive osteolysis due to advanced-stage subungual squamous cell carcinoma.

- **Basal cell tumours**. These arise from germ cells of the skin in the basal layer. Basal cell tumours are the most common tumours in cats (15–16 % of all tumours vs 4–12 % in dogs). They develop late in life (at around 10 years of age in cats and 7–8 years in dogs), and present as solitary, well-circumscribed, solid or cystic masses of varying shapes and sizes. They typically invade the deep dermis and may be alopecic, ulcerated, or pigmented. This last form is the most common in cats. Basal cell tumours occur on the trunk of dogs and on the face, ears, and nose of cats. Surgical excision with deep, wide margins is necessary to prevent recurrence. Basal cell tumours have a low metastatic potential.

Epithelial follicular tumours

Follicular tumours present as firm, solitary, well-circumscribed, and, on occasions, alopecic cutaneous lesions. They mostly show an indolent behaviour and can be resolved by surgical excision.

- **Trichoepithelioma.** Common in dogs.
- **Pilomatricoma.** Common.
- **Trichoblastoma.** Common (Fig. 37).
- **Keratoacanthoma.** Benign keratinocytic lesion in the infundibular area that tends to be filled with keratin.
- **Malignant trichoepithelioma** (malignant epithelioma, follicular carcinoma). Large poorly circumscribed invasive lesion with alopecia and ulceration. Metastases to the skin, vertebrae, and internal organs have been described. En bloc resection is the mainstay treatment.
- **Malignant pilomatricoma** (matricial carcinoma). A very rare tumour found only in dogs. Bone, lung, spleen, and liver metastases have been described. En bloc resection is the mainstay treatment.

Epithelial tumours arising from the sebaceous glands

Most sebaceous gland tumours pursue an indolent course and are easy to manage. They account for 6.8–7.6 % of all cutaneous tumours in dogs and 2.3–4.4 % of those in cats.

- **Sebaceous adenoma.** Tends to affect the head and has a whitish, round, ulcerated appearance (Fig. 38).
- **Sebaceous epithelioma.** A fungiform mass that is normally ulcerated and pigmented. It requires aggressive surgery.
- **Sebaceous carcinoma.** Locally aggressive tumour with the ability to spread to the regional lymph nodes. It typically affects the head. Aggressive surgery is required (Fig. 39).
- **Perianal gland adenoma** (hepatoid gland adenoma). Tumour that arises from modified sebaceous glands in the perianal region. Affects the proximal third of the tail, the lumbosacral region, and the prepuce. These glands are androgen-dependent and are over-represented in male dogs. Perianal gland adenoma accounts for 18 % of all cutaneous tumours in dogs. Cats do not have these glands. It affects dogs aged 8 years or older and typically presents as an ulcerated mass (Fig. 40). Perianal gland adenoma is treated by surgical excision, and in particular, castration (in males), which can result in involution of lesions in 75 % of cases. Oral tamoxifen or deslorelin implants can be used in inoperable cases (Fig. 41).
- **Perianal gland carcinoma** (hepatoid gland adenocarcinoma). A more aggressive tumour with regional and distant involvement. Prognosis is determined by tumour grade, and extensive surgery is required.

Diagnostic interpretation, choice of treatment, and prognosis

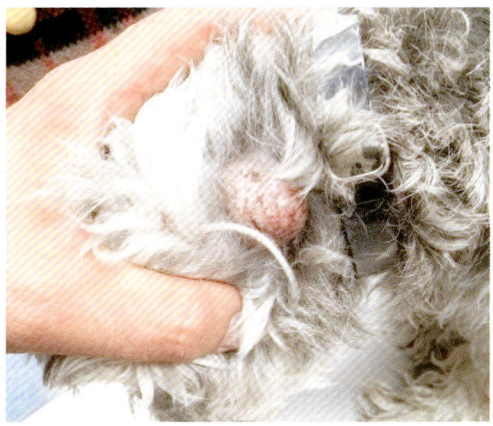

Figure 37. Trichoblastoma on the limb of a dog.

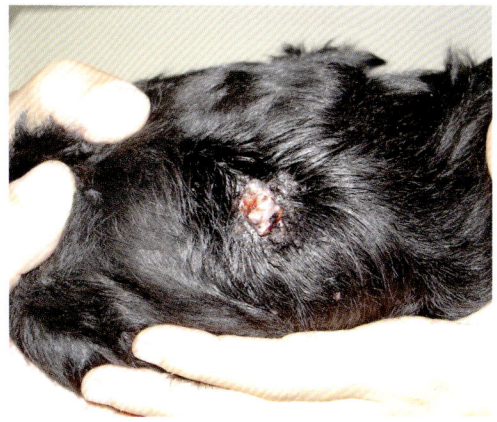

Figure 38. Ulcerated sebaceous gland adenoma.

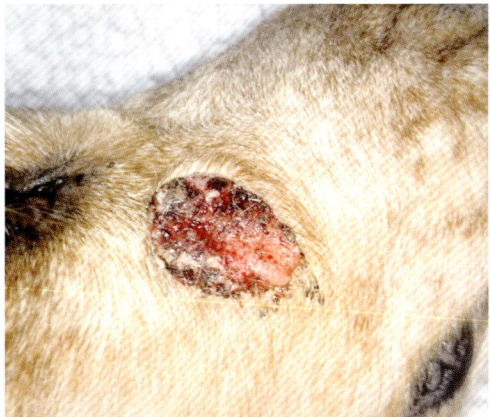

Figure 39. Sebaceous gland adenocarcinoma on the face of a dog.

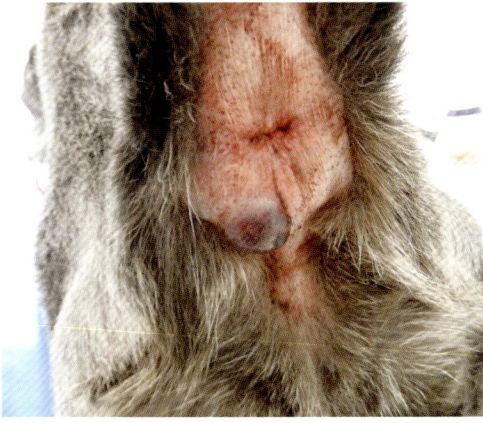

Figure 40. Hepatoid adenoma.

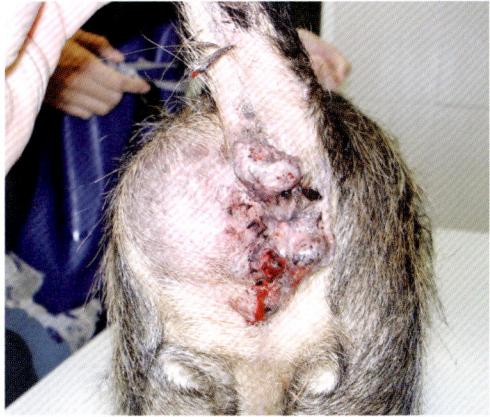

Figure 41. Large, invasive hepatoid adenoma.

Apocrine gland tumours

- **Apocrine cystadenoma, apocrine sweat gland adenoma, and apocrine ductal adenoma.** These tumours are quite similar in terms of presentation and behaviour. They present as firm, fluctuant, cystic lesions, and are treated by surgical excision.
- **Apocrine adenocarcinoma.** Solitary, alopecic, and frequently ulcerated masses that are locally aggressive but have low metastatic potential. Surgical excision with wide margins is the treatment of choice (Fig. 42).
- **Ceruminous gland tumours.** These tumours have a low incidence and are more common in older animals. The presence of a mass in the ear canal can cause otitis. Associated neurological manifestations are seen in 10 % of dogs and 25 % of cats. Malignant variants are more aggressive in cats. They are locally invasive but have a low metastatic potential (10 % in dogs and 15 % in cats at diagnosis) Treatment is surgical (Fig. 43).
- **Apocrine gland adenocarcinoma of the anal sac.** Accounts for 17 % of perianal tumours and just 2 % of cutaneous tumours in dogs. The mean age of presentation is 9–11 years. It is extremely rare in cats. The tumour is normally unilateral and displays highly aggressive local behaviour. Metastasis is also common and affects the regional lymph nodes, lungs, liver, spleen, and bone. Paraneoplastic hypercalcaemia is observed in 25 % of cases and is controlled by surgical excision. Full CT staging is needed due to the high rate of metastasis. The treatment of choice is surgical excision of the primary tumour and affected lymph nodes. Chemotherapy consisting mostly of platinum derivatives can increase survival. Toceranib phosphate has also been used.

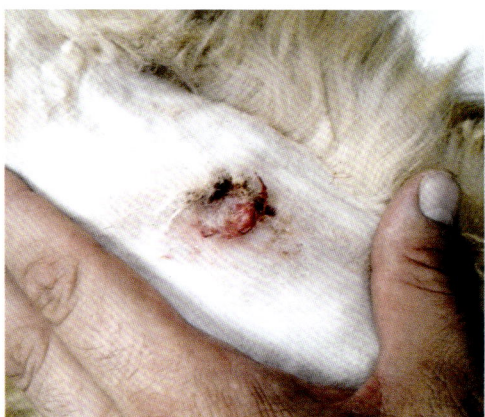

Figure 42. Apocrine adenocarcinoma in a cat.

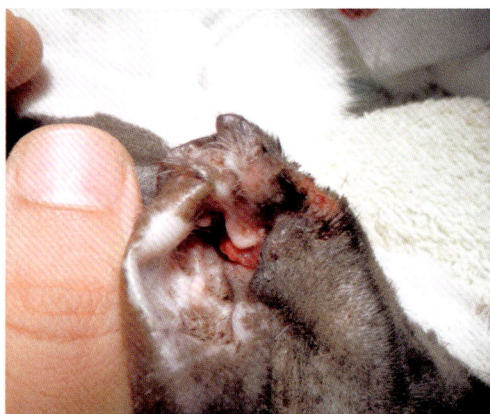

Figure 43. Ceruminous gland adenocarcinoma.

Mesenchymal tumours of the skin

Mesenchymal tumours, and malignant tumours in particular, are relatively common in small animals. This group includes STSs and melanocytic tumours.

Soft tissue sarcoma. The tumours in this group are managed using the same approach as they display similar biological behaviour. Surgical excision with wide margins is the mainstay of treatment and it can be combined with radiation therapy and chemotherapy. Tumour grade is correlated with metastatic potential. The main STSs are:

- **Fibroma.** A benign tumour that is uncommon in both dogs and cats. It presents as a solitary, well-delimited, alopecic mass on the head and limbs.
- **Myxoma.** Similar to fibroma but contains large quantities of mucin.
- **Lymphangioma.** An extremely rare tumour arising in the lymphatic vessels. It presents as large fluctuant masses.
- **Haemangioma.** More common in animals with a white coat and short hair. It is particularly common in the abdominal and inguinal regions and on the inner surface of the limbs as it is induced by ultraviolet radiation. It presents as a well-circumscribed reddish lesion.
- **Lipoma.** A benign tumour that arises in the adipocytes. It presents as a well-delimited soft mass and is common in older dogs with a tendency to be obese.
- **Leiomyoma.** A very rare tumour that occurs on the vulva, perineum, head, and dorsal area.
- **Fibrosarcoma.** A mesenchymal tumour that is more common in the skin and subcutaneous tissue. It accounts for 15–17 % of all cutaneous tumours in cats and 1.5 % of those in dogs. It is the most common ISS in cats. Fibrosarcoma presents as a firm, poorly circumscribed lesion, sometimes with a multilobulated appearance.
- **Myxosarcoma.** A tumour with a fluctuant appearance that contains a viscous fluid.
- **Haemangiosarcoma.** This can present as a dermal or subcutaneous tumour. The dermal variant is more common and has a better prognosis (see section *"Abdominal cavity tumours"*).
- **Haemangiopericytoma.** Exclusive to dogs and seen mostly in elderly animals. It is a low-grade STS.
- **Liposarcoma.** An uncommon tumour with a predilection for the limbs.
- **Leiomyosarcoma.** An uncommon STS.
- **Rhabdomyosarcoma.** A rare tumour that is classified as an ISS in cats. It typically presents as a multilobulated, poorly delimited mass adhered to the deep layers.
- **Nerve sheath tumour** (schwannoma). Similar clinical presentation to haemangiopericytoma.

Melanocytic tumours
- **Cutaneous melanoma.** A mesenchymal tumour that arises in the neuroectoderm. It is relatively common in dogs (5–7 % of all cutaneous tumours) and uncommon in cats (0.8–2.7 %). It affects elderly animals. Unlike melanocytic tumours in other locations (oral cavity, mucocutaneous junction), those involving the skin are largely benign (85 % of cases). However, histopathology is necessary to establish tumour grade, mitotic rate, and lymphatic involvement and hence prognosis. Melanocytic tumours present as small, well-defined, mobile, pigmented lesions (Fig. 44). Fast growth, large size, invasion, ulceration, poorly defined borders, and unpigmented areas are indicative of malignancy. The treatment of choice, surgery, is curative in the majority of cases. Radiation therapy is occasionally used as an alternative.
- **Subungual melanoma.** This is the second most common nail bed tumour. It is associated with regional lymph node metastasis in approximately 50 % of cases, and amputation of the affected digit is the treatment of choice (Fig. 45).

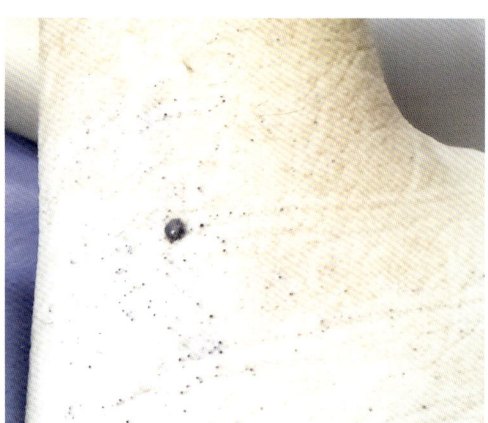

Figure 44. Cutaneous melanoma on the trunk of a dog.

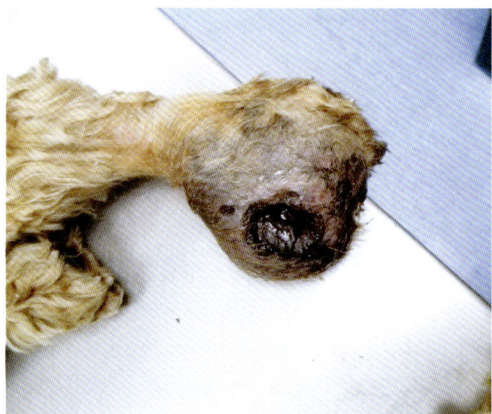

Figure 45. Large subungual melanoma.

Round-cell cutaneous tumours
- **Histiocytoma.** A benign tumour that arises in Langerhans cells. It mainly affects dogs up to 3 years of age, although it can appear at any age. It presents as a fast-growing, solitary, firm, alopecic nodule that can become ulcerated and infected. Histiocytoma is more common on the head and in the front half of the body. Surgical excision is required in the absence of lymphocyte-mediated spontaneous regression.

- **Cutaneous lymphoma.** Accounts for 1 % of cutaneous tumours in dogs and <3 % of those in cats. It is classified as epitheliotropic (located in the epidermis) or nonepitheliotropic (located in the dermis).
  - **Nonepitheliotropic cutaneous lymphoma.** Uncommon in dogs and slightly less so in cats. It occurs as a dermal T- or B-cell infiltrate that can spread to the epidermis and tends to have a multinodular form that spreads quickly. Pruritus is uncommon and there may be hypercalcaemia.
  - **Epitheliotropic cutaneous lymphoma (mycosis fungoides).** This variant is more common in dogs, and particularly in Cocker Spaniels. It is rare in cats. T-cell infiltrate in the epidermis. The clinical manifestations are similar to those seen in skin disorders and range from erythema, inflammation, alopecia, and ulceration to well-defined cutaneous masses or inflammation/ulcers in the oral mucosa. Coexistence of several types of lesions is common. Regional lymph node involvement is common and is followed by spread to distant sites.

  Lymphoma can be diagnosed by cytology, but biopsy is required to determine whether or not the tumour is epitheliotropic. Epitheliotropic LSA is treated with systemic chemotherapy, which can be combined with retinoids. There is evidence of favourable response to masitinib.

- **Cutaneous plasmocytoma.** Accounts for 1.5 % of cutaneous tumours in dogs and is more common in older animals. It is rare in cats. Cutaneous plasmocytoma normally presents as a firm, sessile, solitary lesion that may be alopecic. It affects the ears, lips, digits, face, limbs, trunk, and oral cavity (Fig. 46). Metastasis is rare. The treatment of choice is surgical excision, although radiation therapy has been used in inoperable cases.

- **Cutaneous mast cell tumour.** This is the most common tumour in dogs, in which it accounts for 21 % of all cutaneous tumours. It has a highly variable appearance and is characterised by variations in size due to degranulation processes.

  Multiple lesions have been described, but tumours separated by >5 cm are considered to be independent.

  The mean age of onset is 9 years, and Boxers, French Bulldogs, Pugs, Labrador Retrievers, Golden Retrievers, and Shar Peis are all predisposed. This last breed tends to develop malignant MCTs, which generally appear at a younger age than in other breeds.

  Choice of surgery is determined by tumour grade. Incisional biopsy may be indicated and must be performed with extreme caution to prevent degranulation processes (Fig. 47).

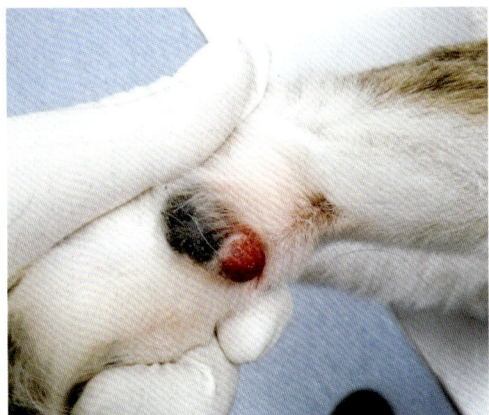

Figure 46. Plasmocytoma on the limb of a dog.

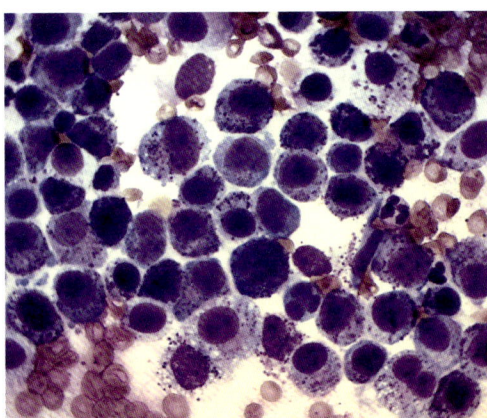

Figure 47. Cytology of a high-grade mast cell tumour.

Regional lymph nodes must be examined by cytology to investigate disease spread. Two systems are used to classify MCTs.
- **The Patnaik system (1984):**
  - Grade I. Round uniform cells containing cytoplasmic granules that can obscure the nucleus. No evidence of mitotic figures. Tumour confined to the dermis.
  - Grade II. Moderately pleomorphic cells with finer and less abundant granules. More variable mitotic rate. Invasion of deeper layers of dermis and subcutaneous tissue. Possibility of necrotic areas or oedema.
  - Grade III. Marked pleomorphism, fewer or even no granules. High mitotic rate. Invasion of deep layers. Necrosis, oedema, and haemorrhage are common.
- **Kiupel 2-tier histological grading system (2011):**
  - Low-grade tumour.
  - High-grade when any of the following criteria are met:
    - ≥7 mitotic figures in 10 high-power (×40 objective) fields (HPF).
    - ≥3 multinucleated cells (≥2 nuclei) in 10 HPF.
    - ≥3 abnormal nuclei in 10 HPF.
    - karyomegaly in ≥10 % mast cells.

Clinical staging is complemented by a complete blood count, an abdominal ultrasound, and hepatic and splenic aspiration. There may also be mild or moderate nonregenerative anaemia due to the presence of gastrointestinal ulcers caused by excessive histamine release. A faecal occult blood test is advisable.

Surgical excision is the treatment of choice for well-circumscribed nonmetastatic MCTs. The surgical approach must be aggressive, with 2-cm lateral margins and one fascial plane deep. Coadjuvant medical treatment must be considered when these margins cannot be achieved.

Chemotherapy is indicated for inoperable, disseminated MCTs and for high-grade MCTs even when adequate safety margins have been achieved.

Chemotherapy regimens are based on prednisone, vinblastine, or lomustine. The use of targeted therapy with tyrosine kinase inhibitors, such as masitinib and toceranib, is opening up new horizons. H_2 antihistamines prevent gastrointestinal ulcers.

Cutaneous MCT in cats is much less common than in dogs, as cats are more prone to visceral MCT. The lesions can be solitary or multiple. There are two forms: **mastocytic**, which is the most common and has similar manifestations to those seen in dogs, and **histiocytic**, which is less common and occurs in young animals. The grading system devised for dogs is not applicable to cats. Treatment is normally surgical.

- **Transmissible venereal tumour (Sticker sarcoma).** This tumour is transmitted through coitus, which explains its high prevalence in rural areas or in areas without routine sterilisation programmes. It affects the external genitalia and the oral and nasal cavities. The tumour has a latency period of 2–6 months. Spontaneous regressions have been described within 3 months of implantation in immunocompetent animals. There have also been reports of metastases to the regional lymph nodes, the skin, bone, spleen, and brain. This tumour is treated with vincristine, which is associated with a complete response rate of 90 %.

Head, neck, and ear tumours

Many of the head, neck, and ear tumours that affect small animals are described in other parts of this book and are therefore just touched on briefly in this section.

- **Carcinomas:** oral SCC (tonsillar SCC is particularly aggressive and has a high potential for regional lymph node and distant metastasis), thyroid carcinoma (neuroendocrine tumour with a tendency to metastasise to the chest), apocrine gland tumours.
- **Sarcomas:** oral FSA, MCT, melanoma.
- **Nasal:** nasal plane SCC, nasal carcinoma, LSA.
- **Brain** (see section "*Nervous system tumours*").
- **Oral cavity:** described in greater detail next.

Oral cavity tumours

Incisional biopsy is usually necessary to make a tentative diagnosis and determine the clinical stage of oral cavity tumours (Table 5). CT scanning is particularly important, as it shows the extent of the tumour and its relationship with other structures. It can also detect regional lymph node involvement and/or distant metastases. The TNM classification system and clinical stages for oral cavity tumours are shown in Tables 6 and 7.

In general, and where feasible, margins of 2–3 cm and >3 cm are recommended for dogs and cats, respectively. Radiation therapy enhances local control in surgery with narrow or "dirty" margins. It is also useful as a palliative treatment when surgery is not an option. Chemotherapy is indicated for tumours with high metastatic potential, despite their low chemosensitivity. Immunotherapy (see Chapter 5) is an option for the multimodal management of oral melanoma.

Table 5. Most common oral cavity tumours in small animals.

	Dog				Cat	
	Melanoma	SCC	FSA	Epulis	SCC	FSA
Percentage	15–20 %	8–15 %	5–12 %	40–50 %	70–80 %	15–20 %
Mean age (years)	12	8–10	7–8	–	10–12	10
Sex	Male	–	Male	–	–	–
Location	Gingiva, labial mucosa	Mandible	Maxilla, hard palate	Mandible	Tongue, pharynx, tonsils	Gingiva
Regional metastasis	40–75 %	<40 % Tonsillar tumours: 73 %	10–30 %		Rare	Rare
Distant metastasis	15–20 %	<35 %	0–70 %	–	Rare	<20 %

Adapted from Lascelles, in *Manual of Canine and Feline Oncology*, BSAVA, 2011.
SCC: squamous cell carcinoma; FSA: fibrosarcoma.

Table 6. TNM classification of oral cavity tumours.

T system (primary tumour)		N system (regional lymph nodes)		M system (metastasis)	
Tis	Carcinoma in situ	N0	No evidence of regional node involvement	M0	No evidence of distant metastasis
T1	<2 cm T1a: without bone invasion T1b: with bone invasion	N1	Movable ipsilateral nodes N1a: without metastasis N1b: with metastasis	M1	Metastasis
T2	2–4 cm T2a: without bone invasion T2b: with bone invasion	N2	Movable contralateral nodes N1a: without metastasis N1b: with metastasis		
T3	>4 cm T3a: without bone invasion T3b: with bone invasion				

Diagnostic interpretation, choice of treatment, and prognosis

Table 7. Stages of oral cavity tumours according to the TNM classification system.

Clinical stage	Definition
I	T1, N0/N1a/N2a, M0
II	T2, N0/N1a/N2a, M0
III	T3, N0/N1a/N2a, M0
	Any T, N1b, M0
IV	Any T, N2b, M0
	Any T, any N, M1

- **Canine oral melanoma** (Fig. 48) is more likely to occur in certain breeds, including Cocker Spaniels, Poodles, Chow Chows, and Golden Retrievers. IHC staining with Melan-A is required to diagnose highly undifferentiated tumours. Oral melanoma is a highly malignant tumour with a high rate of metastasis.
- **Squamous cell carcinoma.** Frequently invades the bone in dogs. Nontonsillar SCC has a low metastatic rate. Risk factors described for cats include the use of flea collars, consumption of tinned food (tuna fish), and exposure to smoke. Lack of local control is a common reason for euthanasia (Fig. 49).

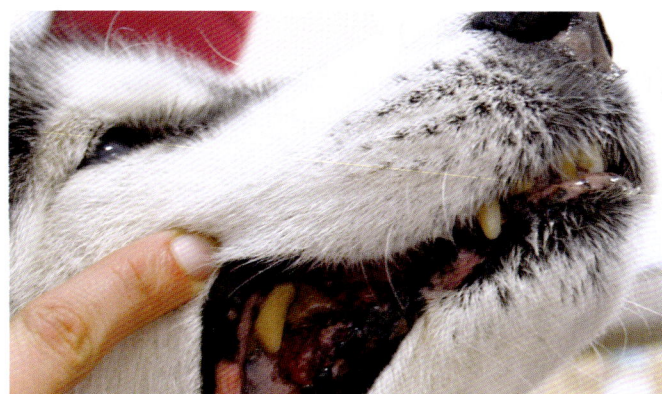

Figure 48. Amelanotic oral melanoma in an 11-year-old male Siberian Husky.

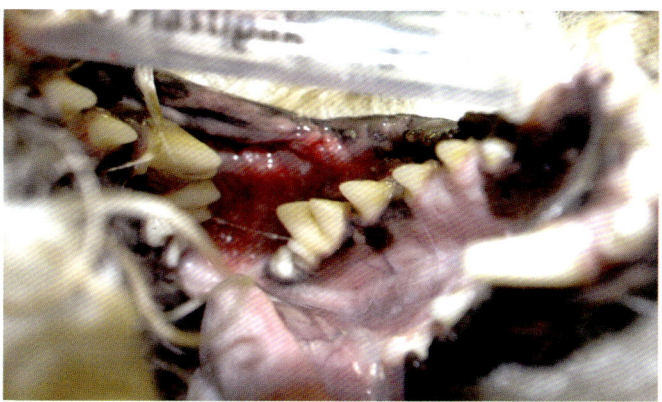

Figure 49. Squamous cell carcinoma in a 13-year-old male Fox Terrier.

- **Fibrosarcoma.** Typical in large breeds (Labrador Retrievers, Golden Retrievers, etc.). It can be difficult to differentiate from a fibroma, but it always displays malignant biological behaviour due to its high recurrence rate (Fig. 50).
- **Epulis.** Benign gum proliferations that arise in the periodontal ligament. They are common in dogs. Noteworthy tumours are ameloblastoma, fibromatous epulis, and ossifying epulis.

The different treatments and prognoses associated with oral cavity tumours are summarised in Table 8.

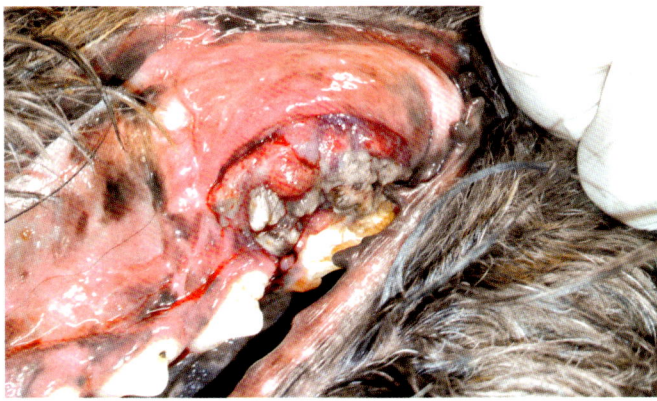

Figure 50. Oral fibrosarcoma in a 10-year-old mixed-breed dog.

Table 8. Treatment and prognosis of oral tumours.

	Dog				Cat	
	Melanoma	SCC	FSA	Epulis	SCC	FSA
Surgery						
Prognosis	Fair	Good	Fair/good	Excellent	Poor	Fair
Recurrence	0–60 %	0–50 %	30–80 %	0–10 %	–	–
Mean survival	5–17 mo	9-26 mo	10–12 mo	>28–64 mo	45 d	–
Survival >1 yr (%)	5–20 %	60–90 %	20–50 %	70–100 %	<10 %	–
Radiation therapy						
Prognosis	Good	Good	Poor/fair	Excellent	Poor	Poor
Mean survival	4–12 mo	16–36 mo	7–26 mo	>37 mo	90 d	–
Survival >1 yr (%)	35-70 %	70 %	77 %	85 %	40 d	–
Treatment of choice	Surgery + radiation therapy/ - immunotherapy	Surgery/ radiation therapy	Surgery/ radiation therapy	Surgery	Surgery + radiation therapy	Surgery/ radiation therapy
Prognosis	Poor/fair	Fair/good	Fair/good	Excellent	Poor	Fair
Death	Distant metastasis	Local/ metastasis	Local	Rare	Local	Local

Adapted from Lascelles, in *Manual of Canine and Feline Oncology*, BSAVA, 2011.
SCC: squamous cell carcinoma; FSA: fibrosarcoma.

Chest cavity tumours
Parenchymal lung tumours

Primary lung tumours are uncommon, but the lung is a preferential site for metastasis from tumours in other locations. The caudal lobe is the most frequently involved location (fig. 51). Clinical signs vary according to location and may include coughing, weight loss, lethargy, and dyspnoea. The tumour might also be detected as an incidental finding. The treatment of choice is surgery combined with chemotherapy. CT examination is therefore necessary before any surgery is planned.

The main primary lung tumours are:
- **Carcinoma:** bronchial, bronchogenic, and bronchioalveolar (most common).
- **Anaplastic carcinoma:** small- or large-cell.
- **Squamous cell carcinoma.**
- **Sarcomas.**
- **Benign tumours** (rare).

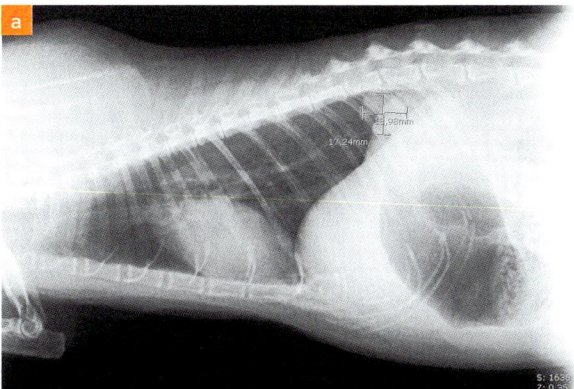
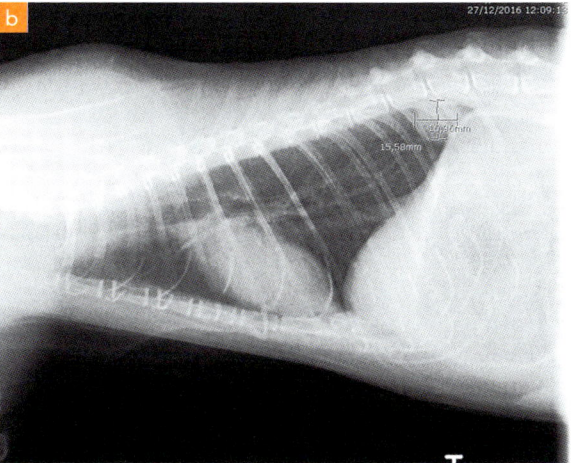
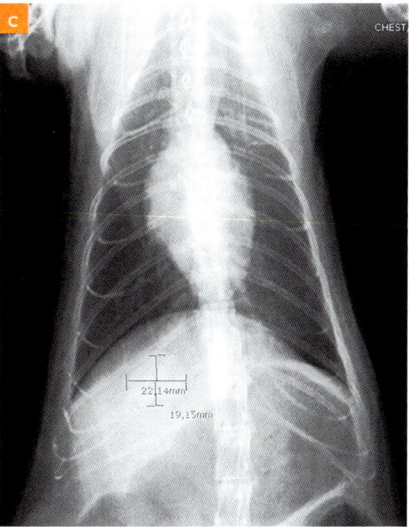

Figure 51. Primary lung carcinoma in a 14-year-old male Persian cat. Note the single mass on the right caudal lobe. Right lateral (a), left lateral (b), and ventrodorsal (c) views.

Cardiovascular tumours

Heart tumours are rare in both dogs and cats. They can be primary or secondary, or intracavitary, intramural, or pericardial. Haemangiosarcoma is the most common primary heart tumour in dogs, followed by chemodectoma (in the aortic body, Fig. 52). Metastasis from LSA is the most common heart tumour in cats. Clinical signs vary according to the size and location of the mass, but the most common finding is cardiac tamponade due to pericardial effusion.

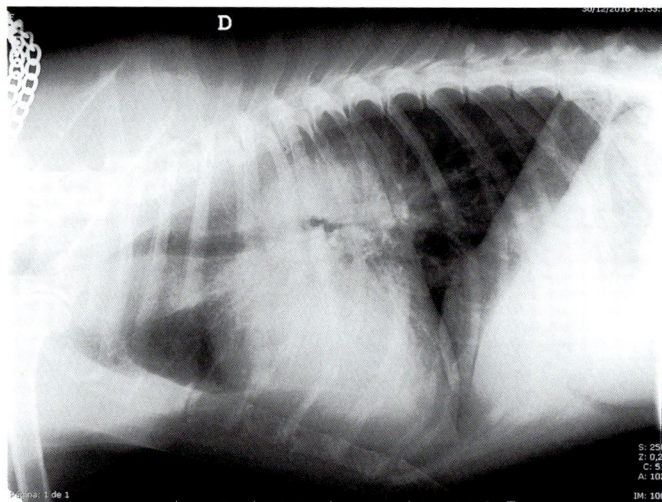

Figure 52. Chemodectoma in the aortic body of a 9-year-old female Rottweiler.

Mediastinal tumours

The mediastinum contains vessels, lymph nodes, the oesophagus, and the thymus. The most common mediastinal tumours are LSAs and thymomas, and again, the clinical signs will vary according to the size and location of the mass. These may include coughing or pleural effusion together with dorsal displacement of the trachea. The treatment of choice will also depend on the nature of the tumour and ranges from chemotherapy (LSA) to surgery (thymoma).

Tumours of the reproductive system
Prostate tumours

One of the main tumours in the reproductive system of small animals is prostate cancer, which has a high tendency to metastasise to the lymph nodes and lumbar vertebrae. It is non-hormone-dependent and extremely rare in cats. Mean survival with chemotherapy (mitoxantrone, carboplatin) is 1–3 months.

Testicular tumours

Testicular tumours are the second most common tumours in male dogs, preceded only by skin tumours. The main types are:

- **Sertoli cell tumour.** This accounts for 50 % of all testicular tumours and presents as a solitary lesion that can measure up to 5 cm. It typically causes atrophy of the contralateral testicle, and there may be feminisation syndrome.
- **Seminoma.** A form of testicular cancer that typically affects testes located in the inguinal area. Less than 10 % of seminomas metastasise to sublumbar or mesenteric lymph nodes or to the spleen or lung.
- **Leydig cell tumour.** Multiple, bilateral tumours with a benign behaviour.

Ovarian and uterine tumours

Ovarian tumours are uncommon (1.5 % in dogs and cats) and are mostly found in elderly animals, with the exception of teratomas, which are associated with a mean age of onset of 4 years. They are normally unilateral, but bilateral tumours have been described. They are mostly carcinomas. They can be asymptomatic or present with vaginal bleeding that progresses to pyometra. The treatment of choice is surgical excision.

Uterine tumours are also uncommon and tend to be myomas (dogs) or endometrial carcinomas (cats).

Tumours can also develop on the vulva or vagina and include myomas, TVTs, carcinomas, and lipomas.

Mammary gland tumours

The management of mammary tumours is complex and beyond the scope of this book. We refer readers to specialised literature on this subject.

As a general rule, however, benign mammary tumours in dogs become malignant with time and should therefore be excised with adequate margins and analysed by biopsy. It was recently shown that castration at the time of mastectomy improved the prognosis of benign tumours and mammary carcinomas. Although there is some debate on this matter, chemotherapy is recommended for advanced clinical stages and grade 2–3 tumours.

Nine out of every 10 mammary tumours in cats are grade III carcinomas. Aggressive surgery is therefore recommended together with, pending consensus, adjuvant chemotherapy.

Abdominal cavity tumours
Canine haemangiosarcoma

Haemangiosarcoma is a malignant tumour that arises in endothelial cells. It accounts for 7 % of all canine tumours. It tends to occur in elderly dogs with a mean age of 10 years, and is more common in German Shepherds, Golden Retrievers, Boxers, and Labrador Retrievers.

With the exception of radiation-induced cutaneous forms, the aetiology of HSA is largely unknown. Radiation-induced lesions occur mainly on the inner thighs, the prepuce, and the ventral surface of the abdomen. Dogs with short hair and light pigmentation are at greater risk.

The main target organ is the spleen (Fig. 53). Haemangiosarcoma accounts for 45–51 % of all splenic tumours, but it can also affect the right atrium (69 % of heart tumours in dogs), the liver, skin, and subcutaneous tissue. It is less common in the lungs, kidneys, oral cavity, bone, bladder, left ventricle, aorta, pulmonary artery, central nervous system, muscle, uterus, and retroperitoneum.

Its biological behaviour is highly aggressive and is characterised by extensive tissue invasion and high metastatic potential. Metastases can occur in any location, but the most common sites are the liver, lungs, peritoneum, lymph nodes, adrenal gland, and diaphragm. Eighty percent of dogs have metastasis (due to haematogenous spread or implantation) at diagnosis (Fig. 54).

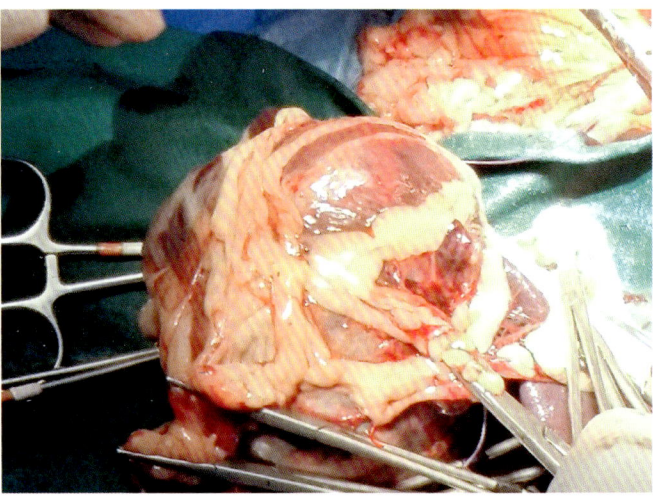

Figure 53. Large splenic haemangiosarcoma.

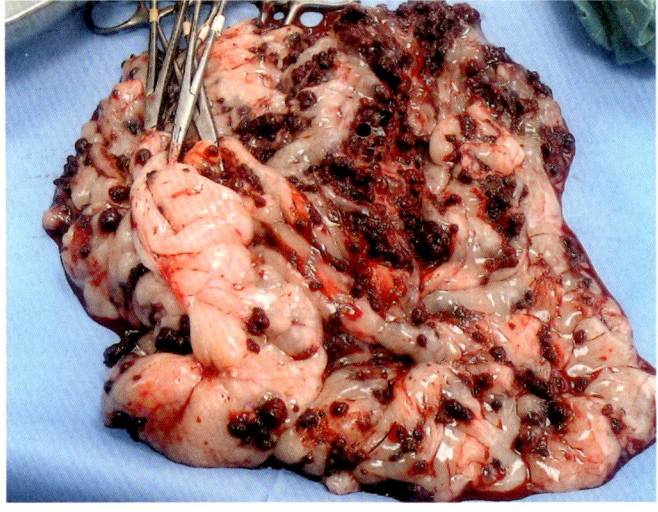

Figure 54. Multiple implantation metastases from a splenic haemangiosarcoma in the omentum.

Diagnostic interpretation, choice of treatment, and prognosis

Characteristics depending on location of haemangiosarcoma

- **Spleen.** Large masses with necrosis and bleeding. These may be solitary or accompanied by smaller lesions. Adherences from old lesions are common. Metastasis is most common in the lungs (miliary or nodular pattern), the liver, and the omentum (Fig. 54).
- **Right atrium.** Metastases largely involving the lungs, spleen, pericardium, subcutaneous tissue, mesentery, intestine, omentum, brain, adrenal glands, peritoneum, and lymph nodes. Haemorrhagic pericardial effusion is common.
- **Skin.** Cutaneous HSA is less aggressive both locally and at a distance than the subcutaneous and muscular forms (Figs. 55–57).

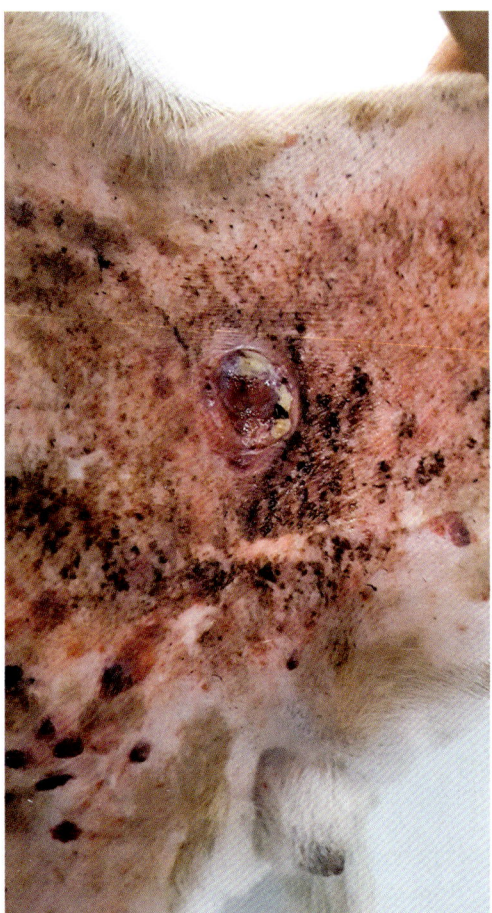

Figure 55. Multiple cutaneous haemangiosarcomas, one of which was deep-seated and ulcerated. Their colour and location on the coat suggest induction by ultraviolet radiation.

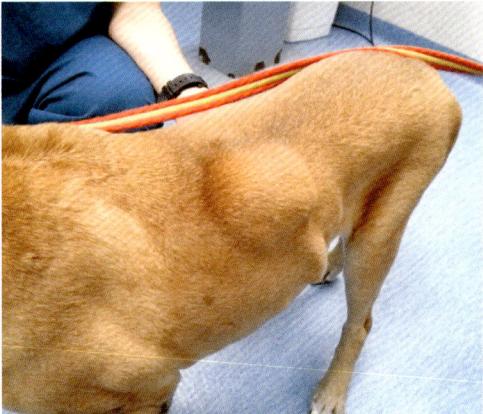

Figure 56. Large subcutaneous haemangiosarcoma.

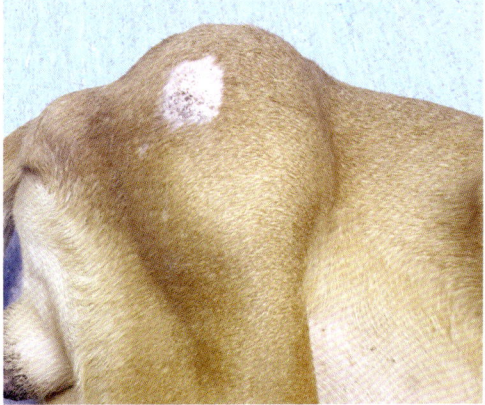

Figure 57. Very advanced muscular haemangiosarcoma.

Forms and clinical signs

Haemangiosarcoma has varying forms. It can appear as solitary or multiple masses affecting one or more organs. It also has varying sizes and appearances, ranging from grey to dark red lesions with a soft to gelatinous consistency. The lesions are poorly circumscribed, nonencapsulated and are normally attached to or invade adjacent structures. They tend to be filled with blood and/or necrotic tissue. Bleeding is also common due to their fragile nature.

The clinical signs of visceral HSA can range from nonspecific signs (apathy, general deterioration, weight loss) to hypovolaemic shock resulting from acute abdominal haemorrhage.

Pets are generally brought for an emergency visit, where supportive treatment (e.g. transfusion) or surgery (e.g. splenectomy) is needed before a definitive diagnosis can be made.

Diagnostic tools

Informative samples contain mesenchymal cells, but cytology is seldom diagnostic. Histopathology is needed for a definitive diagnosis, but this can also be complicated by bleeding and necrosis, which may cause confusion with a haematoma. In such cases, IHC staining with CD31 and von Willebrand factor (WF) (Fig. 58) is necessary.

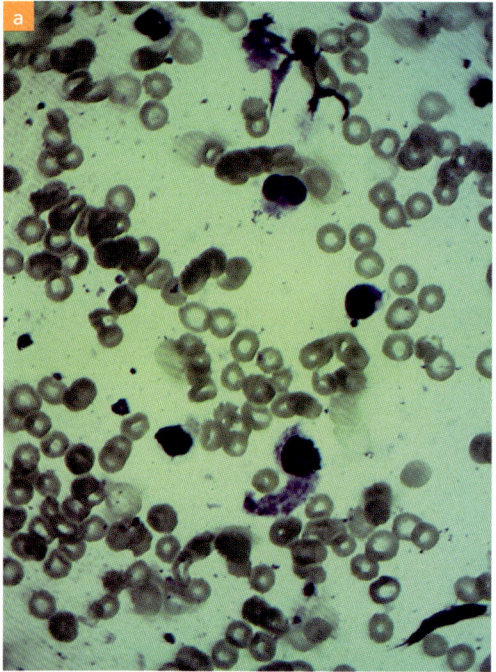
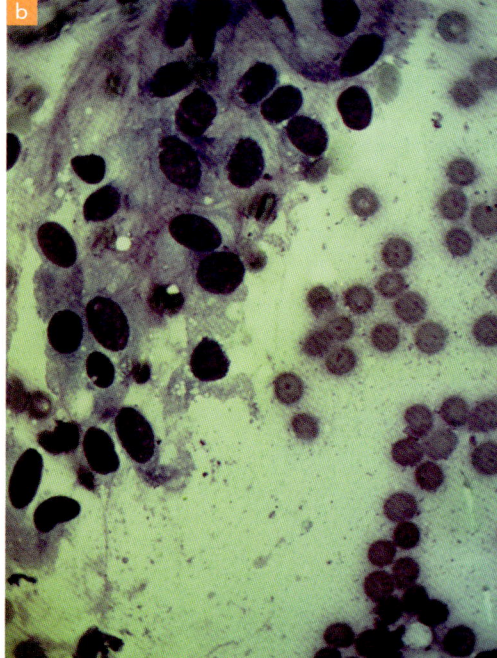

Figure 58. Cytology of a haemangiosarcoma.

Clinical staging in HSA requires the following tests:
- A complete blood count. In most cases, this shows anaemia (regenerative or nonregenerative depending on the time of diagnosis), neutrophilia, and severe thrombocytopenia (Fig. 59). The blood smear will show nucleated erythrocytes, schistocytes, and acanthocytes (Fig. 58b).
- Coagulation tests. Approximately 50 % of cases have associated disseminated intravascular coagulation, which, in turn, is associated with a mortality of 25 %.

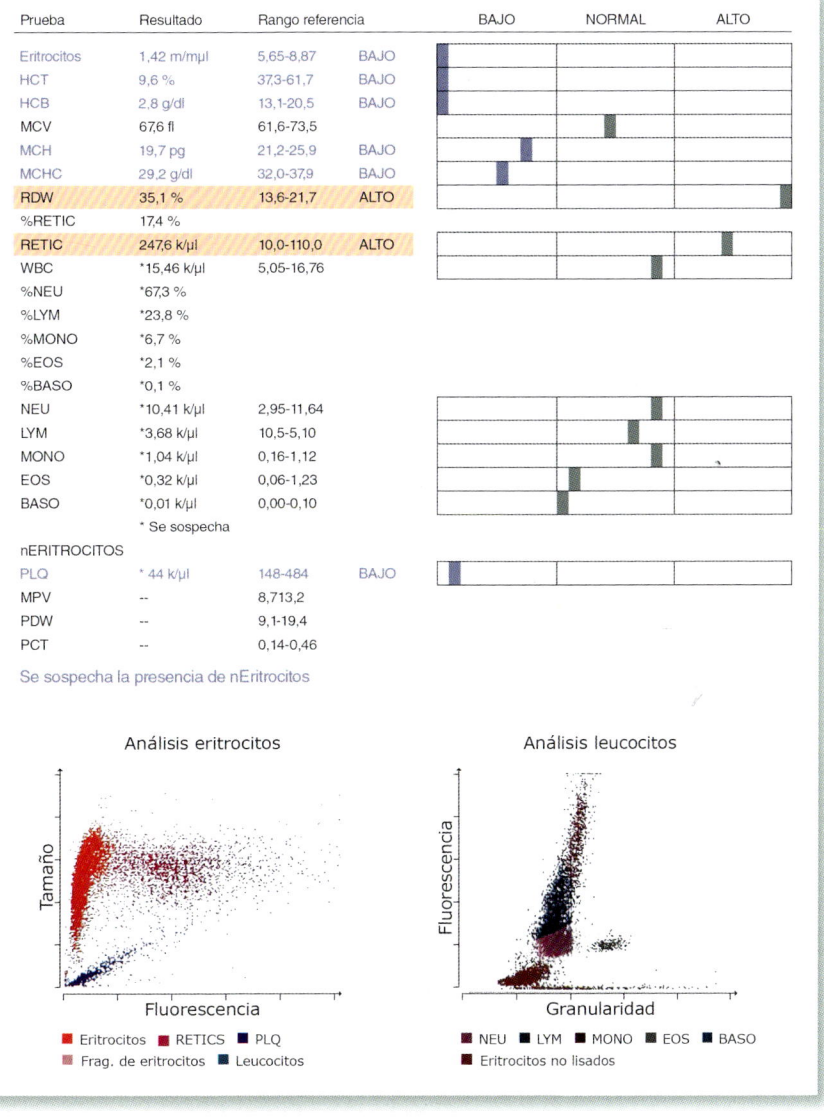

Figure 59. Example of complete blood count results for a haemangiosarcoma associated with severe highly regenerative anaemia, thrombocytopaenia, and nucleated erythrocytes.

- Chest radiography. Three projections are needed to rule out metastasis and identify possible pericardial effusion or a mass at the base of the heart. The X-rays may not show the metastases, but they will show associated pulmonary haemorrhage (Figs. 60 and 61).
- Abdominal ultrasound. Abdominal masses and haemorrhages.
- Heart ultrasound. Pericardial effusion or intracardial masses. Failure to detect a mass on an ultrasound scan does not mean that it does not exist.
- Advanced imaging techniques (CT and MRI) can help to establish clinical stage (Figs. 62–64).

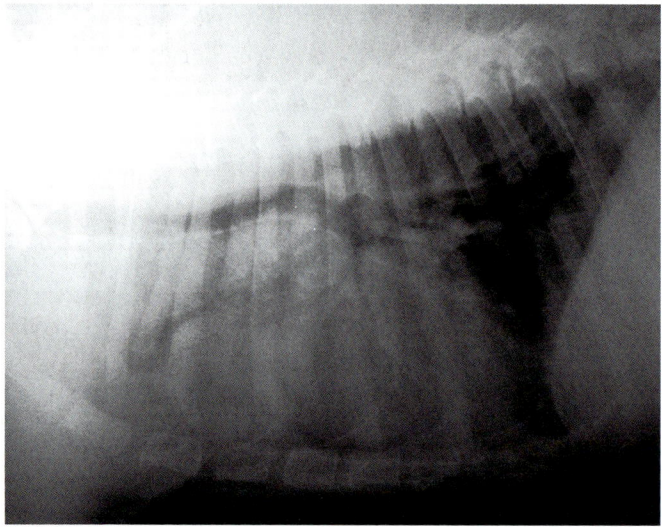

Figure 60. Large pulmonary metastasis from a subcutaneous haemangiosarcoma.

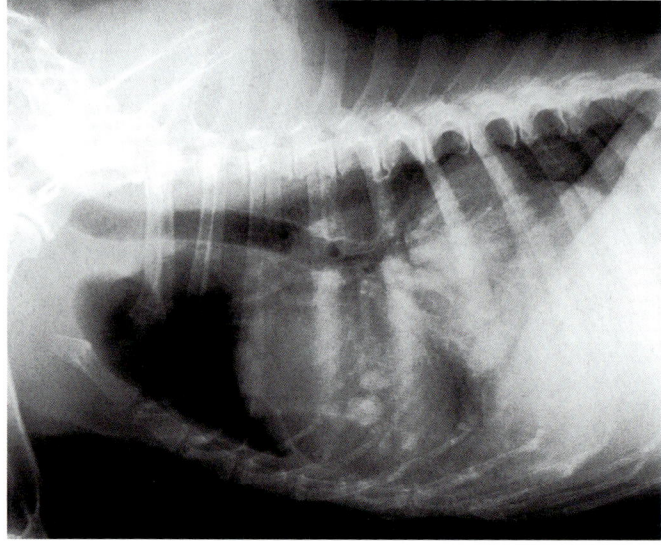

Figure 61. Multiple lung metastases from a splenic haemangiosarcoma.

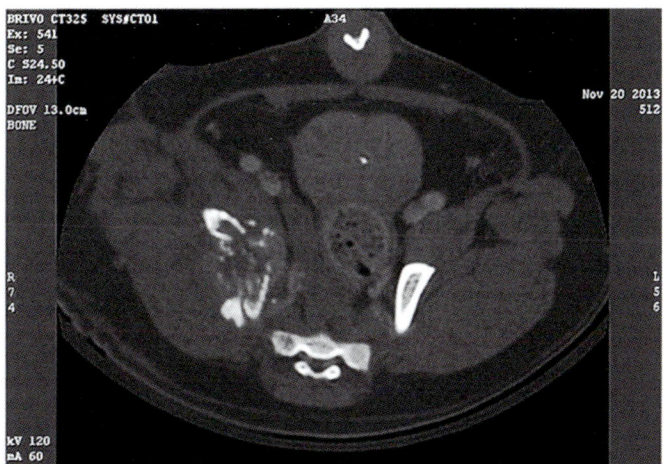

Figure 62. CT image of a pelvis showing major bone destruction by a bone haemangiosarcoma.

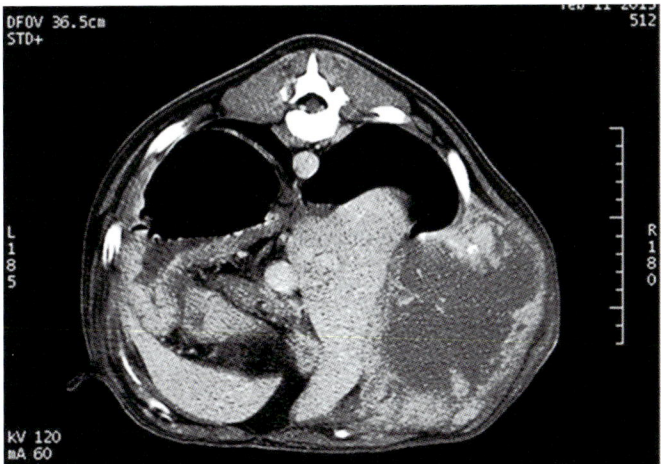

Figure 63. CT image of a large rib mass ultimately diagnosed as a rib haemangiosarcoma.

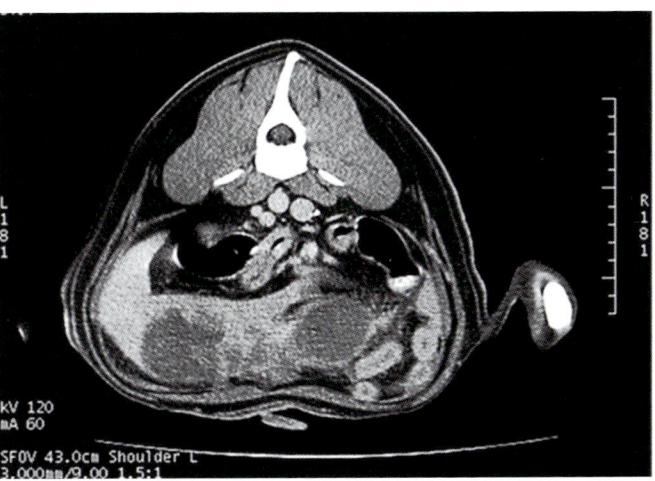

Figure 64. CT image of splenic masses in the patient in Figure 63.

The TNM system used for canine HSA is shown in Tables 9 and 10.

Table 9. TNM classification system for haemangiosarcoma.

T system primary tumour		N system N Regional lymph nodes		M system Metastasis	
T0	No evidence of tumour	N0	No lymph node involvement	M0	No evidence of distant metastasis
T1	<5 cm confined to the primary site	N1	Involvement of regional lymph nodes	M1	Distant metastasis detected
T2	>5 cm or broken, with invasion of subcutaneous structures	N2	Involvement of distant lymph nodes		
T3	Tumour invasion of adjacent structures, including muscle				

Table 10. Clinical stages of haemangiosarcoma (HSA) according to the TNM classification system.

Clinical stage	Visceral HSA	Cutaneous HSA
I	T0/T1, N0, M0	Lesions confined to the dermis
II	T1/T2, N0/N1, M0	Lesions affecting the subcutaneous tissue
III	T2/T3, N0/N1/N2, M1	Invasion of underlying muscle

Treatment and prognosis

The treatment of choice is surgery, although patients often need to be stabilised first. Survival in patients with splenic HSA treated with surgery only is 19–86 days (<10 % of patients survive for 12 months).

In patients with heart involvement, manifestations can be controlled by pericardiocentesis and pericardiectomy.

Cutaneous and subcutaneous forms require surgical treatment similar to that used for STS, i.e. lateral margins of approximately 2 cm and one fascial plane deep. Prognosis is better in cutaneous HSA (up to 987 days with surgical treatment only). The subcutaneous variant requires adjuvant chemotherapy (mean survival of 425 days vs 175 for surgical treatment only and 64 for chemotherapy only).

Haemangiosarcoma is sensitive to doxorubicin and therefore the first-line chemotherapy regimens are based on doxorubicin (as monotherapy), VAC (vincristine, doxorubicin, cyclophosphamide), or AC (doxorubicin, cyclophosphamide) (see Appendix II). Where contraindicated (see Chapter 5), doxorubicin can be replaced with epirubicin.

Metronomic therapy achieves survival rates similar to those seen with traditional chemotherapy.

Digestive tumours

- **Stomach.** Stomach tumours are uncommon. Of note in this category are gastric carcinoma in dogs and LSA in cats. Clinical manifestations are slow to appear and are nonspecific (gastritis). They include weight loss and, in the case of carcinoma, signs of chronic bleeding due to ulcers. Diagnosis requires imaging tests (ultrasound, CT) and the collection of samples by endoscopy or laparotomy. The treatment of choice is surgery combined with chemotherapy (doxorubicin, toceranib) in the case of carcinoma and systemic chemotherapy in that of LSA.
- **Intestine.** Intestinal tumours other than LSA are uncommon. Most cases are malignant (carcinomas, leiomyomas, gastrointestinal stromal tumours [GISTs], MCT) and are more common in the small intestine of cats and the large intestine of dogs. Clinical signs are uncommon and depend on anatomical location. The main intestinal tumours are:
    - **Carcinoma.** This tumour normally shows signs of intestinal stenosis/obstruction and can affect any part of the intestinal tract in dogs. In cats, it tends to affect the jejunum and the ileum. It metastasises to the mesenteric lymph nodes, liver, lungs, peritoneum, spleen, kidneys, and pericardium.
    - **Lymphoma.** Jejunum in dogs and ileum in cats. Involvement of the regional lymph nodes and even the kidneys and liver is common at diagnosis.
    - **Visceral mast cell tumour.** Rare in dogs and relatively rare in cats. There tends to be metastasis to the spleen, lymph nodes, and liver at the time of diagnosis. Biopsies of the full thickness of the tumour is recommended, as visceral MCT tends to affect the muscle. The treatment of choice is surgery with margins of 5–10 cm.
- **Liver.** Liver tumours are more often malignant in dogs and benign in cats. While the liver is a site for metastasis from certain tumours, it is also home to primary tumours within four major groups:
    - **Hepatocellular carcinoma.** Nodular hyperplasia, hepatocellular adenoma, and hepatocellular carcinoma (HCC). There are three types of HCC:
        - Massive: large solitary mass confined to a single liver lobule.
        - Nodular: multifocal, involving several lobules.
        - Diffuse: multifocal or converging tumours affecting all liver lobules.
    - **Bile duct cancer** (cholangiocellular adenoma and carcinoma).
    - **Neuroendocrine or carcinoid tumours.**
    - **Mesenchymal tumours.**

There is no specific breed or sex predisposition and the mean age of onset is 10 years. Diagnostic imaging techniques are essential and must include chest radiography, abdominal ultrasound, and even CT, particularly when surgery is being contemplated. Ultrasound-guided sample collection for cytology or biopsy is a very useful diagnostic tool, although prior coagulation profiles are recommended as the procedure causes bleeding complications in approximately 5 % of cases. Up to 60 % of cytological examinations and 90 % of biopsies are diagnostic.

Prognosis depends on histological subtype and is favourable following the surgical excision of benign tumours and massive HCC. Massive HCC tends to present as a solitary liver lobule, favouring surgical excision. In addition it has low to moderate metastatic potential (0–37 %) and therefore has a better prognosis than either nodular or diffuse HCC, in which complete surgical excision is generally not possible. These tumours also have high metastatic potential (93 % and 100 %, respectively). It is not known whether nodular and diffuse HCCs are metastases from a primary HCC.

They must be distinguished from neoplastic lesions, such as hyperplastic or regenerative nodules.

- **Pancreas.** Pancreatic tumours can be primary (adenoma, adenocarcinoma) or secondary. Most primary exocrine pancreatic tumours are carcinomas and account for <0.5 % of all tumours in dogs and cats. Pancreatic carcinomas are very aggressive. They normally originate in the ductal system, but they can also arise from the acini.

  Insulinoma is an endocrine pancreatic tumour characterised by periods of hypoglycaemia with concomitant hyperinsulinaemia. Other causes of hypoglycaemia must be ruled out before establishing a tentative diagnosis of insulinoma. The treatment of choice is surgery.

Urinary tract tumours

- **Kidneys.** Kidney metastases are more common than primary kidney tumours and they are accompanied by signs of chronic kidney disease, with or without kidney failure. The following tumours are possible:
  - Carcinomas:
    - Renal carcinomas: these show a predilection for male dogs and affect the renal cortex, with invasion of the vena cava and metastases to the lymph nodes, liver, lungs, brain, and bone.
    - Transitional cell carcinoma (TCC) or SCC: affect the renal pelvis.
  - Lymphoma: more common in cats.
- **Bladder.** Malignant tumours (TCC, SCC, or other carcinomas) are more common than benign tumours (fibroma, leiomyoma, or papilloma) in the bladder, and they normally affect dogs. They generally cause lower urinary tract signs.

Diagnostic interpretation, choice of treatment, and prognosis

There are four patterns of TCC: papillary, nonpapillary, infiltrative, and noninfiltrative. The tumours are fast-growing and spread rapidly to the regional lymph nodes. Transitional cell carcinoma can be spread by implantation and cytology samples should therefore not be collected by cyst puncture. In addition, extreme care should be taken if surgery is performed. Surgery must be combined with chemotherapy (mitoxantrone or chlorambucil).

Nervous system tumours

Nervous system tumours have numerous distinctive features.
- They are inaccessible in terms of collecting cytology or biopsy samples.
- Their clinical signs vary considerably according to location and include, among others, mood disorders, vestibular syndromes (central or peripheral), seizures, trembling, ataxia, circling, head pressing, paraparesis, monoparesis, tetraparesis, hemiparesis, blindness, facial paralysis, and muscle group atrophy.
- Treatment is complicated by the blood–brain barrier.

There are no specific classification systems for nervous system tumours in veterinary medicine. In 2007, the World Health Organization (WHO) updated the system for classifying tumours of the CNS in humans (Table 1), and this is extrapolated for use in small animals. Nervous system tumours are also classified according to their anatomical location, as this has a determining impact on clinical signs and treatment options (e.g. possibility of surgery).
- Brain tumours
  - Intra-axial or extra-axial (Fig 65).
  - Supratentorial or infratentorial.
- Medullary tumours
  - Intramedullary.
  - Intradural-extramedullary.
  - Extradural.

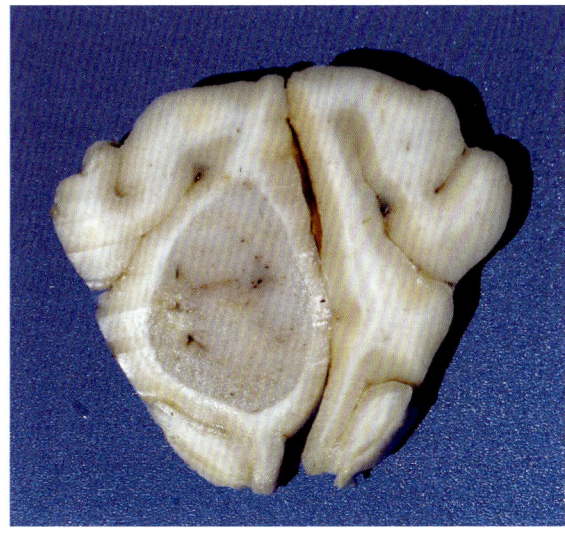

Figure 65. Well-delimited intra-axial tumour on the front right lobe of a Boxer.

Veterinary neuro-oncology has made great strides in recent years, mainly thanks to advances in diagnostic imaging and treatment options (e.g. radiation therapy, surgery, and stereotactic biopsy).

Table 11. Histological classification of tumours of the nervous system in domestic animals.

1. Neuroepithelial tumours	1.1. Astrocytic tumours	1.1.1. Low-grade (well differentiated) astrocytoma	1.1.1.1. Fibrillary
			1.1.1.2. Protoplasmic
			1.1.1.3. Gemistocytic
		1.1.2. Medium-grade astrocytoma (anaplastic)	
		1.1.3. High-grade astrocytoma (glioblastoma)	
	1.2. Oligodendroglial tumours	1.2.1. Oligodendroglioma	
		1.2.2. Anaplastic (malignant) oligodendroglioma	
	1.3. Other gliomas	1.3.1. Mixed glioma (oligoastrocytoma)	
		1.3.2. Gliosarcoma	
		1.3.3. Gliomatosis cerebri	
		1.3.4. Spongioblastoma	
	1.4. Ependymal tumours	1.4.1. Ependymoma	
		1.4.2. Anaplastic (malignant) ependymoma	
	1.5. Choroid plexus tumours	1.5.1. Choroid plexus papilloma	
		1.5.2. Choroid plexus carcinoma	
	1.6. Neuronal and mixed neuronal-glial tumours	1.6.1. Gangliocytoma	
		1.6.2. Ganglioglioma	
		1.6.3. Olfactory neuroblastoma (esthesioneuroblastoma)	
	1.7. Embryonal tumours	1.7.1. Primitive neuroectodermal tumour (PNET)	1.7.1.1. Medulloblastoma
			1.7.1.2. PNETs, excluding cerebellar origin
		1.7.2. Neuroblastoma	
		1.7.3. Ependymoblastoma	
		1.7.4. Thoracolumbar spinal cord tumour of young dogs (nephroblastoma)	
	1.8. Pineal parenchymal tumours	1.8.1. Pineocytoma	
		1.8.2. Pineoblastoma	

2. Tumours of the meninges	2.1. Tumours of the meningothelial cells[1]	2.1.1 Meningioma	2.1.1.1. Meningotheliomatous
			2.1.1.2. Fibrous (fibroblastic)
			2.1.1.3. Transitional (mixed)
			2.1.1.4 Psammomatous
			2.1.1.5. Angiomatous (angioblastic)
			2.1.1.6. Papillary
			2.1.1.7. Granular cell
			2.1.1.8. Myxoid
			2.1.1.9. Anaplastic (malignant)
	2.2. Mesenchymal, non-meningothelial tumours	2.2.1. Fibrosarcoma	
		2.2.2. Diffuse meningeal sarcomatosis	
3. Lymphosarcoma and hematopoietic tumours	3.1. Lymphosarcoma		
	3.2. Non-B, non-T leukocytic neoplasm (neoplastic reticulosis)		
	3.3. Microgliomatosis		
	3.4. Malignant histiocytosis		
4. Tumours of the sellar region	4.1. Suprasellar germ cell tumour		
	4.2. Pituitary adenoma		
	4.3. Pituitary carcinoma		
	4.4. Craniopharyngioma		
5. Other primary tumours and cysts	5.1. Vascular hamartoma		
	5.2. Epidermoid cyst		
	5.3. Pituitary cyst		
	5.4. Other cysts		
6. Metastatic tumours			
7. Local extensions of regional tumours	7.1. Nasal carcinoma		
	7.2. Multilobular tumour of bone		
	7.3. Chordoma		
8. Tumours of the peripheral nervous system	8.1. Ganglioneuroma		
	8.2. Peripheral neuroblastoma		
	8.3. Paraganglioma		
	8.4. Peripheral nerve sheath tumour	8.4.1. Benign (schwannoma, neurofibroma)	
		8.4.2. Malignant (malignant schwannoma, neurofibrosarcoma)	

[1] All slow-growing except the anaplastic variants. In people they are classified as grade I (psammomatous, transitional, meningothelial, and fibroblastic, grade II (atypical and choroid), and III (anaplastic and papillary) according to the indications of the WHO. Grade II tumours have not been identified in cats.

Intracranial tumours

Intracranial tumours are much more common in dogs than cats (2.6–4.5 % vs 0.0035–2.2 %).

While they can affect dogs and cats of any age, they are more common in adults (mean age of 9 years). Brain tumours are the second most common neoplasm in young animals, preceded only by haematopoietic tumours. The most common types are medulloblastomas (Fig. 66), epidermoid cysts, and teratomas, although meningiomas have been described in cats <3 years and in dogs <6 years.

Intracranial tumours have no specific sex predisposition. They do, however, show a predilection for certain breeds, in particular, Boxers and Golden Retrievers, followed by Scottish Terriers, Bobtails, Boston Terriers, French Bulldogs, and Rat Terriers. Finally, brachycephalic breeds are more likely to develop gliomas and pituitary tumours, while dolichocephalic breeds, especially those weighing >25 kg, are at greater risk of meningiomas. No breed-specific predisposition has been identified in cats.

Clinical signs can appear suddenly or progressively, and owners frequently attribute early signs (loss of vision, limb weakness, or disorientation) to ageing or other causes. Onset of signs depends on the location of the tumour, its growth rate, and the presence of other conditions, such as peritumoural oedema, brain haemorrhage, obstructive hydrocephaly, and cerebral hernia.

Seizures occur in 50 % of dogs and 23 % of cats, and together with mood changes, are the most common clinical sign. The most common signs in cats are changes in states of consciousness, circling, seizures, and general deterioration.

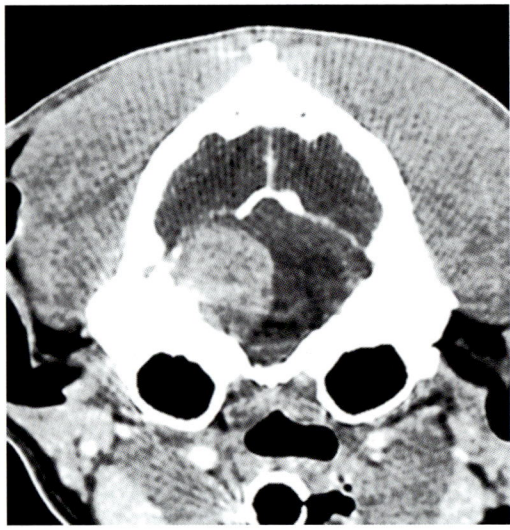

Figure 66. Cross-sectional CT image of a medulloblastoma in a Labrador aged 1.5 years.

Spinal cord and peripheral nerve tumours

Spinal cord tumours are the second most common cause of myelopathy in cats (after inflammatory or infectious lesions). The most common spinal cord tumour is LSA (39 %), followed by OSA (16 %).

Spinal cord tumours cause different degrees of limb weakness, and on occasions, pain. Clinical signs tend to progress faster in intramedullary tumours than in extradural tumours. Neurological signs can appear suddenly due to oedema, ischaemia, infarction, or haemorrhage.

Peripheral nerve tumours tend to cause lameness (frequently interpreted as an orthopaedic or neuromuscular problem) that progresses to monoparesis (Fig. 67) and causes muscular atrophy of the affected limb and pain.

Medullary tumours can be extradural, intradural–extramedullary, intramedullary, or mixed.
- **Extradural tumours.** These are the most common tumours in dogs and cats and can be bone tumours (OSA/osteoma, FSA/fibroma, chondrosarcoma/chondroma), HSA, multiple myeloma, liposarcoma/lipoma, carcinoma, or LSA (this last tumour is more common in cats). They may also be metastases from other tumours.
- **Intradural–extramedullary tumours.** These include meningiomas, nerve sheath tumours (schwannomas, neurofibromas, neurofibrosarcomas), and thoracolumbar spinal cord tumours in young dogs (nephroblastoma). Nerve sheath tumours can affect any of the peripheral nerves (including the cranial nerves). They strictly belong to the peripheral nervous system.

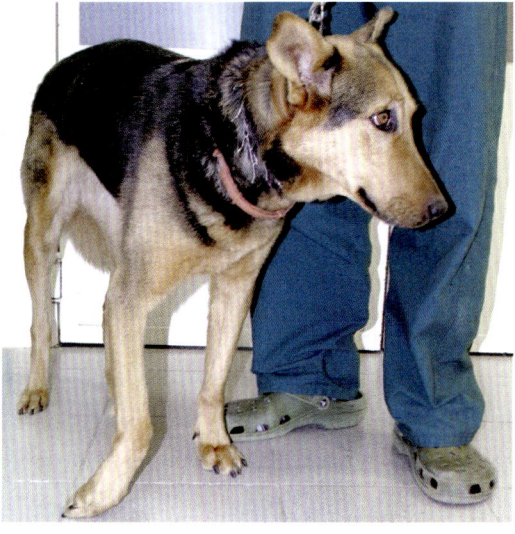

Figure 67. Monoparesis and muscular atrophy (more evident on palpation) due to a nerve root tumour.

- **Intramedullary tumours.** Astrocytomas, oligodendrogliomas, ependymomas, and metastases.
- **Mixed-compartment tumours.** Peripheral nerve sheath tumours and LSA.

The following tests are needed to locate tumours: a myelograph (with two views), a simple CT scan, a myelo-CT scan, and MRI (which provides greater precision for evaluating intramedullary lesions).

Benign tumours resemble malignant tumours because of their location and clinical manifestations.

Brain tumours induce angiogenesis and the newly formed vessels lack a blood–brain barrier, facilitating the transfer of water to brain tissue (vasogenic oedema).

Pituitary tumours tend to be associated with endocrine-related disorders.

Diagnostic procedure

The main components of the diagnostic procedure for nervous system tumours are:
- **Blood tests.** These rule out metabolic, toxic, or inflammatory disorders as the origin of clinical signs. The results are generally normal.
- Brain or spine **X-rays.** These are of limited diagnostic value.
- **Cerebrospinal fluid** (CSF). The results of CSF analysis are generally normal or nonspecific, but tumour cells may be seen with certain tumours, such as choroid plexus tumours, gliomas, and histiocytic sarcomas.
- **Chest X-rays.** Metastases are very rare.
- **Advanced imaging techniques.** The diagnostic tool of choice is MRI (Figs. 68 and 69). There is a close relationship between MRI findings and histological subtype (Table 12). In gliomas, for example, the degree of contrast uptake is significantly associated with tumour grade. Necrosis and cysts are also more common in high-grade tumours. Angiographs combined with MRI or CT are used to assess tumour vascularity prior to surgery and/or interventional embolisation.

- **Monitoring of lesions.** Repetition of imaging studies is of value for determining the biological behaviour of lesions (with or without medical treatment).
- **Stereotactic biopsy.** Minimally invasive CT- or MRI-guided biopsy.
- **Histopathology study.** Definitive diagnostic tool for determining tumour type and grade.

Table 12. MRI characteristics of brain tumours.

MRI characteristic	Explanation
General characteristics of tumours in dogs and cats in T1 and T2	Hypointense and isointense in T1 and hyperintense in T2. Granular cell tumours are often hyperintense in T1. This is also the case with 20 % of meningiomas.
Contrast uptake	Most brain tumours take up contrast. More common in high-grade gliomas than in low-grade tumours due to microvascular proliferation.
Oedema	Peritumoural hyperintensity in T2. More common in astrocytomas than in oligodendrogliomas and in rostrotentorial than in infratentorial meningiomas. Tends to be particularly severe in granular cell tumours (rare).
Cystic structures	These can appear in all types of tumours, but are more common in meningiomas (25 %).
Dural tail sign	Typically seen in meningiomas, but also in other diseases.
Ring-like sign	Typically seen in gliomas, but also in other diseases.

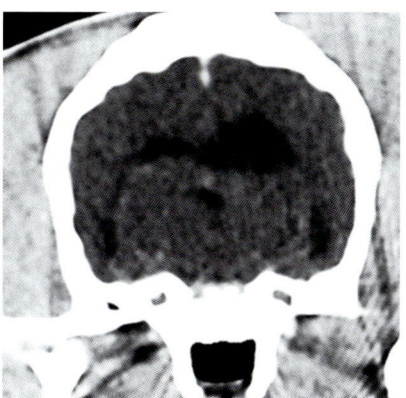

Figure 68. Cerebral asymmetry with a mass effect in the right thalamus; the origin could not be identified by CT.

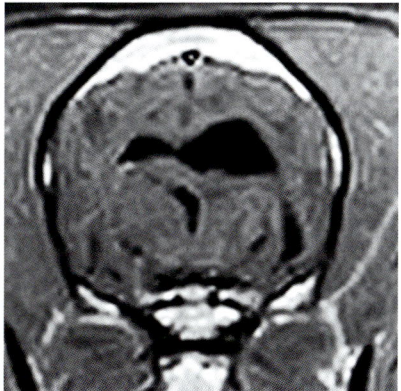

Figure 69. MRI can rule out a tumour (as it is the most sensitive technique for nervous system lesions).

Treatment of nervous system tumours

The main treatments in nervous system tumours are:
- **Corticosteroids.** Very effective at reducing associated vasogenic oedema. They also reduce vascular endothelial growth factor expression. The recommended protocol is oral prednisone 0.5 mg/kg/12 h for 14 days, followed by 0.5 mg/kg/24 h for another 14 days and 0.5 mg/kg/48 h indefinitely.
- **Anticonvulsants.** The anticonvulsant of choice is phenobarbital, although caution is necessary as this drug can alter the metabolism of corticosteroids and other chemotherapeutic agents through the induction of cytochrome P-450. Phenobarbital produces sedation in 70 % of patients, and some authors recommend using levetiracetam or zonisamide instead.
- **Cyclooxygenase-2 inhibitors.** The use of selective cyclooxygenase 2 (COX-2) inhibitors in this setting appears to be justified by the overexpression of COX-2 in human meningiomas. This isoenzyme, however, has not been found to be expressed in canine or feline meningiomas.
- **Progesterone.** Sex hormone receptors have been observed in a large number of canine and feline meningiomas.
- **Chemotherapy.** Temozolomide has been used in humans. In dogs and cats, hydroxyurea, lomustine, and nitrosyl cobalamin have all been used, but with varying results.
- **Tyrosine kinase inhibitors.** No studies have demonstrated the effectiveness of tyrosine kinase inhibitors in dogs or cats with nervous system tumours.
- **Intrathecal chemotherapy.** Used in human medicine to treat intracranial and medullary tumours and acute lymphoblastic leukaemia in children. No safety and efficacy studies have been conducted in dogs.
- **Surgery.** Surgery, sometimes combined with radiation therapy, is the treatment of choice for nervous system tumours. Different surgical approaches are used depending on the location of the tumour and the material used for excision.
  - **Ventriculoperitoneal shunting.** The insertion of a ventriculoperitoneal shunt can achieve temporary resolution of clinical signs in tumours blocking CSF drainage. Stabilising the patient prior to biopsy, craniotomy, or radiation therapy helps.
  - **Craniotomy in meningiomas.** Craniotomy in this setting is associated with an immediate postoperative mortality rate of 19 % in dogs and 17 % in cats, in addition to complications such as pneumocephalus and pneumorrhachis in dogs and blindness, anaemia, and acute kidney injury in cats. Surgery combined with radiation therapy achieves the best survival outcomes in meningioma. In 20 % of cats, tumours recur over a mean period of 9.5 months. Seizures disappear in 50 % of cases of meningiomas treated with surgery and radiation therapy. Surgical resection can be

complicated by several factors, including the location of the tumour, the absence of a clear line between the tumour and the surrounding healthy tissue, invasion of healthy parenchyma, and tumour friability (Fig. 70).
- **Endoscopic surgery.** This option is associated with a shorter recovery time and is particularly useful for tumours that are difficult to access. According to one study, the mean survival time for dogs with meningiomas treated with endoscopic excision was 5.8 years.
- **Ultrasound aspiration.** One study of dogs with meningiomas observed longer survival with ultrasound aspiration than with traditional surgery, even when this was combined with radiation therapy.

- **Radiation therapy.** There are two therapeutic modalities for radiation therapy:
  - Radiation therapy for brain tumours: total dose of 45–54 Gray (Gy) (2.5–3 Gy per session) over 3–4 weeks.
  - Palliative radiation therapy: 38 Gy (5–9 Gy per session) over 5 weeks.
  - Stereotactic radiation therapy (radiosurgery): 25–30 Gy in 1–5 sessions. This technique requires lower anaesthetic doses and is associated with less damage to healthy tissue and minimal adverse effects.

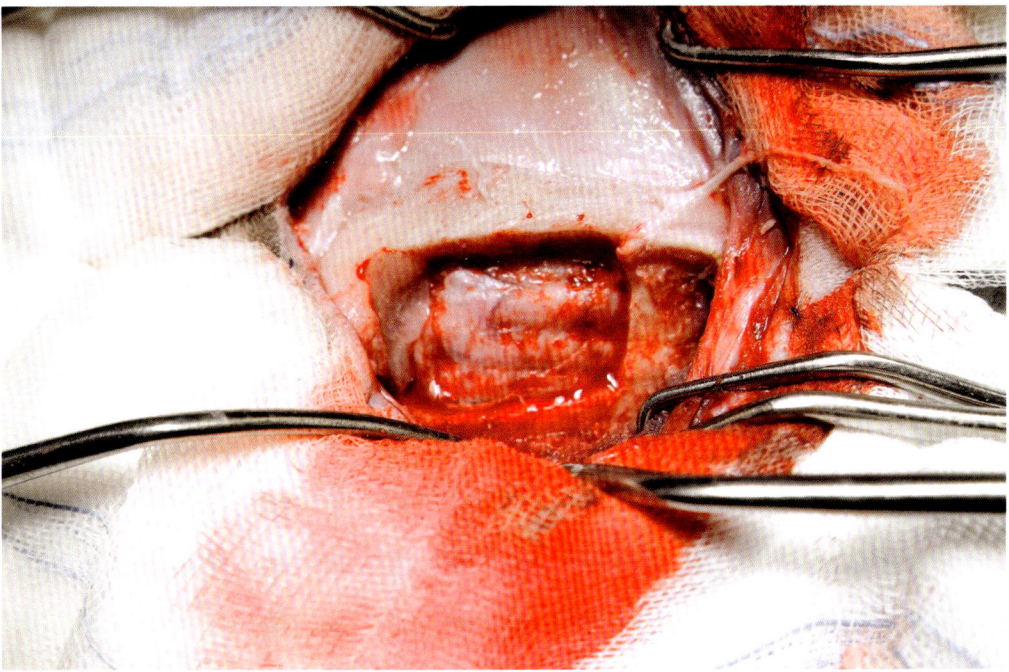

Figure 70. Rostrotentorial craniotomy. The location of the tumour determines the approach and possible postoperative complications.

Few studies have analysed survival in patients with histopathologically confirmed tumours treated using the same modality. Location is also an important survival factor, but tumours of the same type can vary greatly in terms of location. Supratentorial tumours, for example, are associated with a 4-fold longer survival than infratentorial tumours ("the more cranial a tumour, the better"). Mean survival of patients treated palliatively (with corticosteroids, anticonvulsants) is 30–90 days (Appendix IV).

Skeletal tumours

Bone tumours are relatively common in small animals and are even more common in dogs. Osteosarcoma accounts for 85 % of all malignant bone tumours. Other bone tumours (excluding haematopoietic tumours) are chondrosarcoma, FSA, HSA, and histiocytic sarcoma.

Osteosarcoma

Canine OSA affects large and giant breeds, and 75% of these tumours develop in the appendicular skeleton. The most common sites are the proximal humerus, distal radius, distal femur, and proximal tibia. Bone tumours involving the forelimbs are twice as long as those involving the rear limbs and generally affect the metaphysis of the long bones. The rest develop in the axial skeleton: mandible (27 %), maxilla (22 %), cranium (14 %), ribs (10 %), nasal cavity (9 %), and pelvis (6 %) (Figs. 71 and 72). Finally, a small percentage of OSAs are extraosseous (Fig. 73).

The tumours can be proliferative and/or lytic. They rarely affect other bones, and metastasis via haematogenous spread is very common and mainly affects the lungs (Fig. 74). There may be spontaneous fractures (Fig. 75).

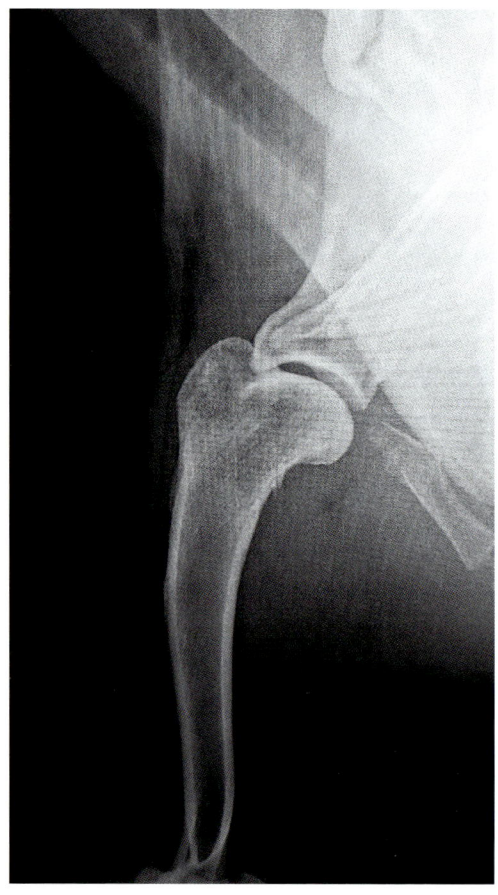

Figure 71. Osteosarcoma on a humeral head.

Diagnostic interpretation, choice of treatment, and prognosis

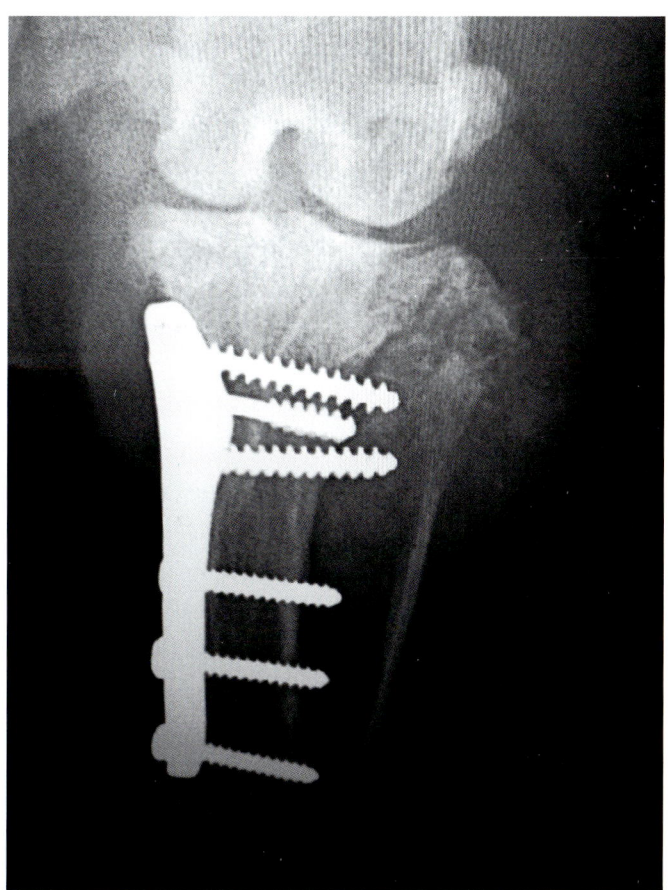

Figure 72. Osteosarcoma in the fibula of a dog with a fracture fixation implant in the tibia; osteosarcoma associated with the fixation implant.

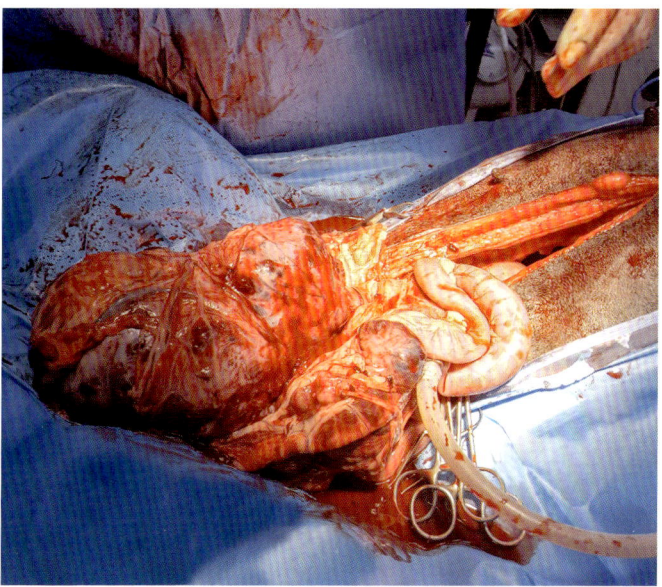

Figure 73. Atypical form of high-grade osteosarcoma in the omentum extending into the intestine and spleen.

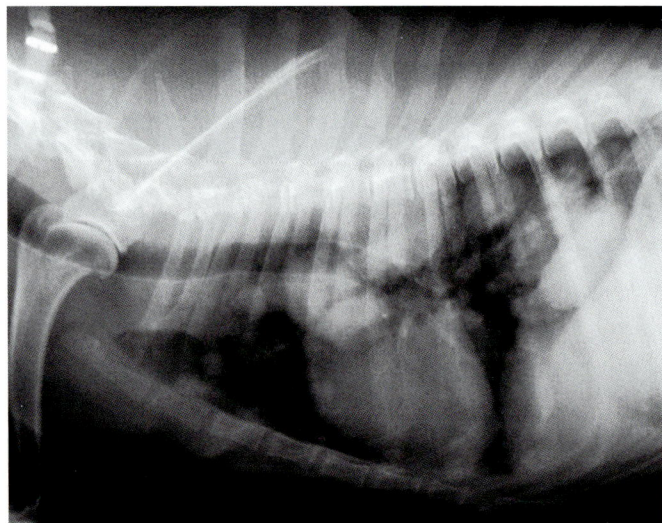

Figure 74. Lung metastasis in an osteosarcoma.

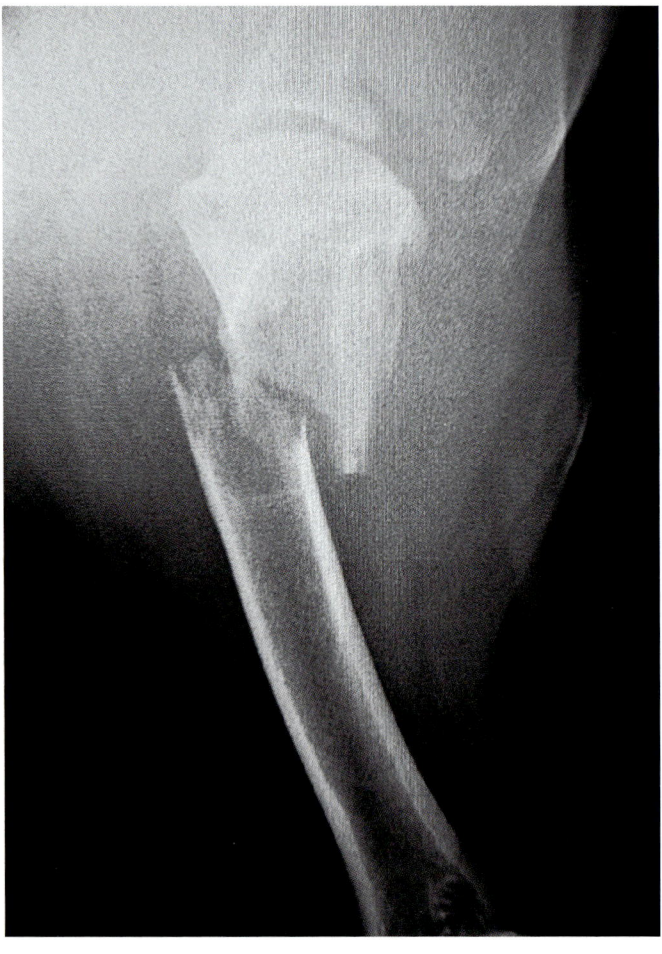

Figure 75. Spontaneous fracture caused by osteosarcoma in the proximal humerus.

Ultrasound-guided cytology is used to diagnose tumours in lytic areas. If the results are not diagnostic, an incisional biopsy with a Jamshidi needle or an excisional biopsy is needed. Samples must be taken from the lesion and not from the transition zone between the tumour and healthy tissue. Prognosis is linked to tumour grade, location, age, and increased levels of alkaline phosphatase.

Treatment is surgical and frequently requires amputation of the limb followed by chemotherapy (with carboplatin, doxorubicin, or a combination of both).

Chondrosarcoma

Chondrosarcoma is the second most common tumour in dogs (10 % of all bone tumours), and shows a predilection for flat bones (nasal cavity, ribs).

The life expectancy for patients with costal chondrosarcoma is approximately 1000 days after radical excision (of the affected rib and two adjacent ribs). To date, there have been no studies demonstrating the effectiveness of chemotherapy. Patients tend to die following metastatic spread, which occurs in the late stages of disease.

Bone haemangiosarcoma

Primary HSA can affect the bones or muscles. It is locally aggressive and has high metastatic potential (Figs. 76 and 77).

The standard treatment is surgery followed by chemotherapy with doxorubicin or chemotherapy as monotherapy.

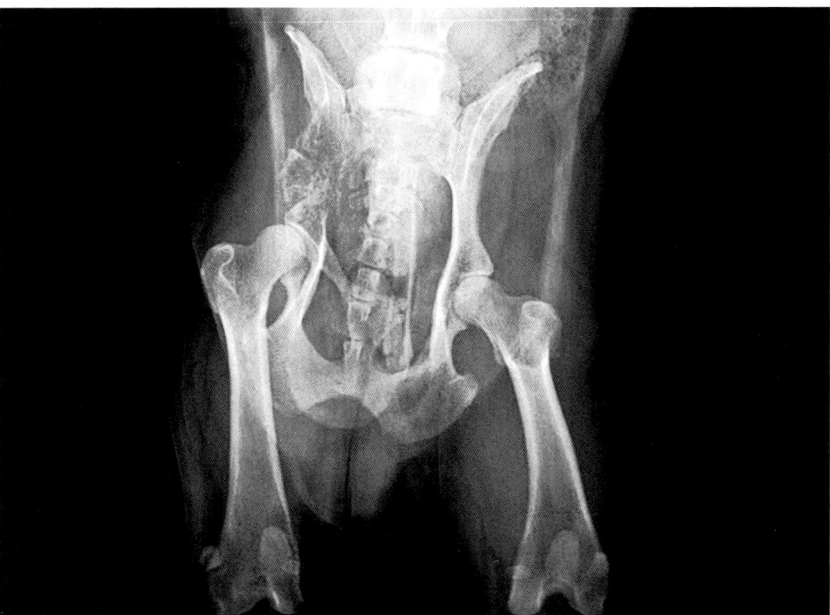

Figure 76. X-ray of an osseous haemangiosarcoma in the ileum.

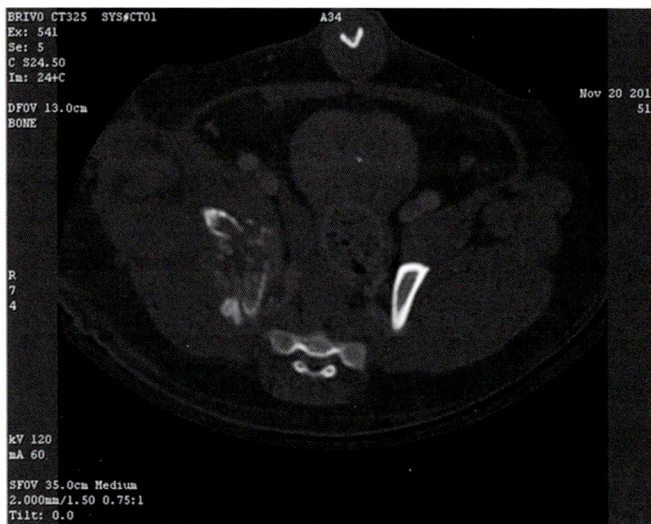

Figure 77. CT image of the same lesion as in Figure 76.

Fibrosarcoma
Fibrosarcoma can be difficult to distinguish from OSA if the samples are poorly representative. The treatment of choice is surgery (amputation) and risk of metastasis is determined by tumour grade.

Multilobular osteochondrosarcoma
Uncommon tumour that affects the cranial bones. The radiographic image of this tumour is highly characteristic as it shows a "popcorn" pattern. Potential for late metastasis. Where feasible, tumours should be removed surgically.

Synovial sarcoma
Malignant joint tumour with a moderate rate of metastasis to the lungs and lymph nodes (20–50 %). Prognosis is determined by tumour grade, clinical stage, and treatment. The treatment of choice is amputation. No role has been defined for chemotherapy in synovial sarcoma.

Histiocytic sarcoma
Histiocytic sarcoma can only be distinguished from synovial sarcoma using IHC staining, but the distinction is important as both management and prognosis vary considerably. It can present as periarticular or disseminated disease (worse prognosis). High metastasis rate. Treatment is based on radical surgery and chemotherapy (lomustine).

Bone metastases

Bones are a relatively common site for metastases from tumours that spread through the blood (higher incidence of urogenital tumours, mammary tumours, and anal sac adenocarcinoma). The most common sites of involvement are the ribs, pelvis, lumbar vertebrae, and the humerus and femur (where involvement of the diaphysis is more common) (Fig. 78).

Haematopoietic tumours

Haematopoietic tumours constitute an extremely complex group of tumours and we will mention just two types:
- Those that arise in the bone marrow: leukaemia, MM, myeloproliferative disorders.
- Those that arise in the lymphatic system: LSA, bone marrow metastases (MCT, carcinomas).

See section *"Hematopoietic tumours"* in *"Biological behaviour of tumours according to tissue of origin"*

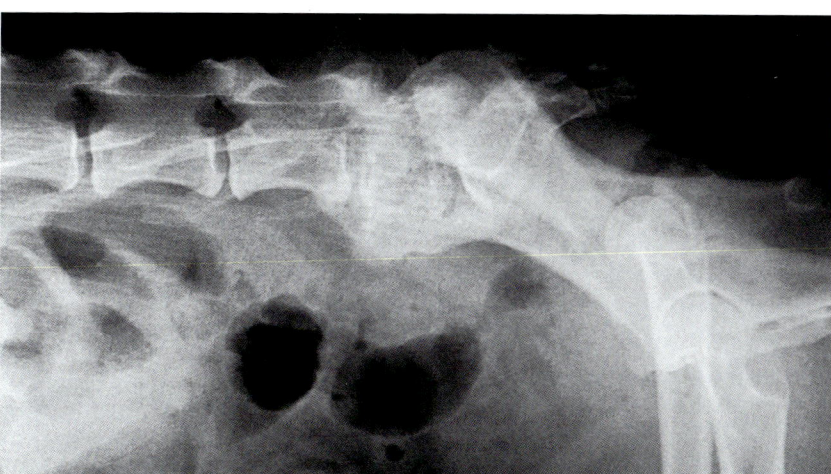

Figure 78. Vertebral metastasis from an apocrine gland adenocarcinoma of the anal sac.

ADVANCED-STAGE TUMOURS

Treating a patient with an advanced-stage tumour is perhaps one of the greatest challenges facing a veterinary surgeon, as it is necessary to determine whether or not the patient is still enjoying a good quality of life, and if not, to advise the owners that the time has come to "let go".

Veterinary surgeons must be objective in such cases and guide the owner through this difficult time. Antiangiogenic treatments have revolutionised the management of advanced-stage tumours in patients with an adequate quality of life.

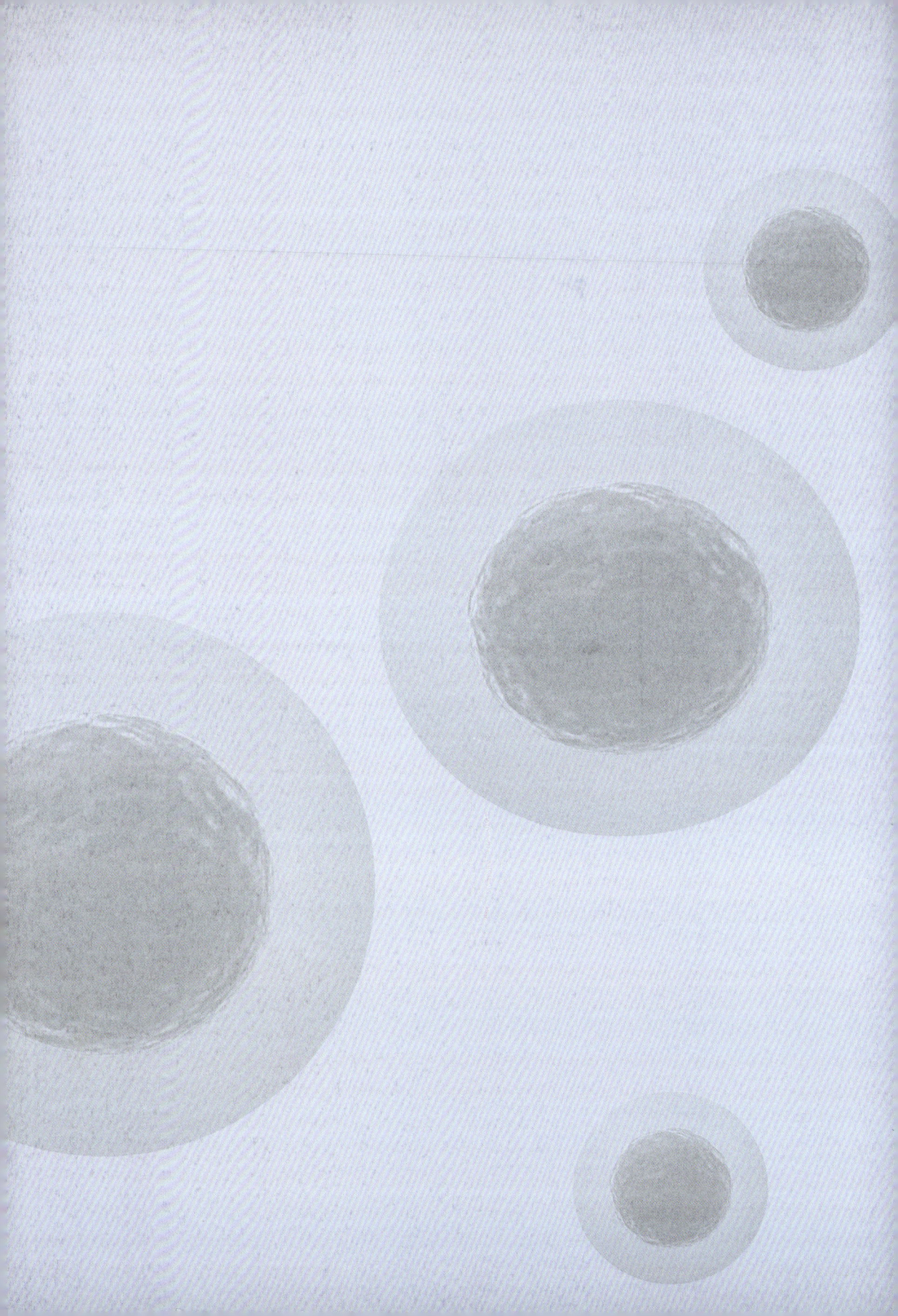

5

Cancer treatment

The greatest challenge in veterinary oncology is treating patients with concomitant conditions. The pillars of cancer treatment are surgery, chemotherapy, and radiation therapy. Surgery is generally (but not always) the best option. However, it is not always feasible and in some cases, it is not even an option (e.g. in lymphosarcoma or leukaemia). In all cases, it is necessary to contemplate the patient's age, ability to recover, quality of life, and life expectancy. Before deciding on any treatment, it is necessary to determine the **biological behaviour** of the neoplasm.

Surgery

Introduction

Surgery is the treatment of choice for solid tumours. Its effectiveness depends on the patient's general health, lifestyle, and activity, on the type and stage of tumour being treated, and on the possibility of (or need for) adjuvant therapy.

Surgery can be used in isolation or form part of a complex treatment protocol including radiation therapy or chemotherapy. Age, breed, sex, and weight can all be determining factors when planning surgery.

- **Age.** Age alone is not a negative prognostic factor, but the presence of age-related diseases can influence a patient's prognosis or ability to recover.
- **Sex, species, and breed.** In some cases, these factors can influence clinical presentation and biological behaviour. These, in turn, will determine how aggressive the surgical approach should be. A cutaneous mast cell tumour, for example, is much more aggressive in Shar Peis than in other breeds.
- **Weight and physical health.** Both overweight and poor physical health can complicate surgery.

Oncology surgeons must be trained in anatomy, physiology, and excision and reconstruction techniques. They must also be familiar with the biological behaviour of the tumour in question and with the existence of alternative or complementary treatments in order to offer the best possible solution. In addition, they must weigh up the risks and benefits of each option and be familiar with the risks of functional or cosmetic impairment.

From a practical perspective, the **chances of achieving a cure are greatest in the first operation**. In such cases:
- The lesion is surrounded by healthy tissue that facilitates the surgeon's work.
- The peripheral areas of the tumour are the most active and vascularised areas and must be properly removed.

- Subsequent operations are undertaken in newly created anatomical planes, and this requires a more aggressive surgical approach, which results in smaller volumes of healthy tissue to heal and hence greater difficulties in ensuring complete excision (Figs. 1 and 2).

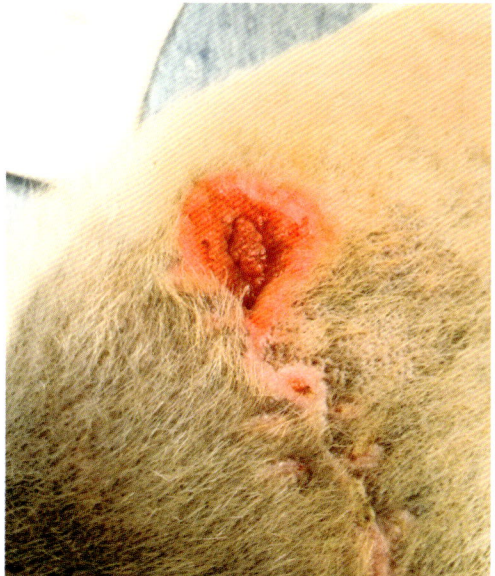

Figure 1. Soft-tissue sarcoma that recurred following excision without adequate margins.

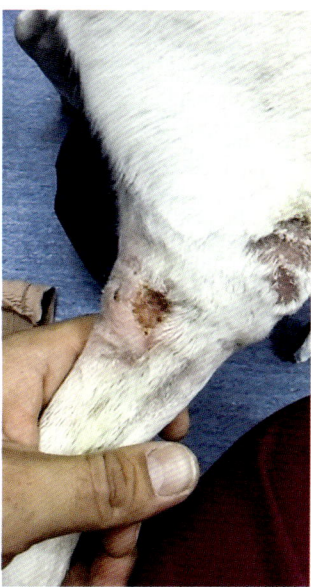

Figure 2. Recurrence of a limb mast cell tumour excised without adequate margins.

Surgeons need to know the measurements of the mass in advance to plan the safety margins accordingly. Margins must be measured in fresh, not formalin-fixed tissue (fixation reduces margins by 35–42 %). It is therefore essential to carefully label the surgical margins before fixation (e.g. with sutures or Indian ink) for subsequent laboratory analysis.

While diagnostic imaging techniques are often needed to plan surgery, surgeons must also carefully palpate all lesions and examine the surrounding areas and regional lymph nodes. They should also be familiar with the patient's diagnosis (informed by cytology or biopsy) and with the clinical stage and biological behaviour of the tumour. Finally, many tumours have a capsule or pseudocapsule that also needs to be removed.

Indications

Oncological surgery forms part of the diagnostic and treatment workup. It is thus a necessary component of biopsy sample collection, curative surgery, palliative surgery aimed at relieving local clinical signs, and cytoreduction prior to chemotherapy or radiation therapy.

Sample collection
Incisional biopsy. This involves collecting a fragment of the mass using needle biopsy (Tru-cut), punch biopsy, or incisional wedge biopsy (with a scalpel). The use of electrosurgical pencils is contraindicated, as they cause coagulation.
Excisional biopsy. This procedure involves the complete removal of the mass. It is contraindicated for fast-growing masses, masses with poorly defined margins, oedema, local erythema, or ulceration, injection-site sarcoma (ISS), mast cell tumour (MCT), soft tissue sarcoma (STS), and haemangiosarcoma (HSA).

Therapeutic surgery
The main determinants of surgical success are the experience of the surgeon, tumour type and location, clinical stage, and species (excision of an MCT, for example, requires a more aggressive approach in dogs than in cats or ferrets).

In all cases, cytology and biopsy tracts must be removed together with an adequate margin of healthy tissue. This must be done by en bloc excision, with rapid ligation of vessels in order to minimise the release of tumour emboli during manipulation of the tumour.

The mass must be managed gently to avoid spread of the tumour to the surgical bed. This is done by separating it from the surgical field and avoiding contact with other areas. Different gloves, gauze, and surgical instruments must be used when excising the tumour and when closing the wound to prevent the transfer of neoplastic cells (Figs. 3–5).

There are four categories of surgical excision:
- Intracapsular. The mass is removed in different blocks through debulking. Surgery with margins is not possible in this case.
- Partial or marginal. The mass is removed from just outside the capsule or pseudocapsule. The procedure leaves residual microscopic disease (Fig. 6).
- Wide. This involves complete excision of the mass together with healthy surrounding tissue (Fig. 7).
- Radical. The entire structure or body compartment is removed (e.g. in amputation), resulting in the elimination of all traces of residual disease (Fig. 8).

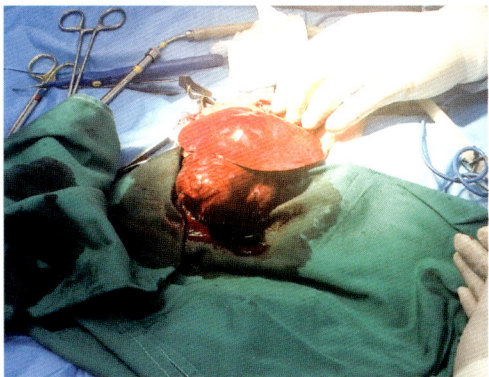

Figure 3. Abdominal masses must be separated from other organs before excision.

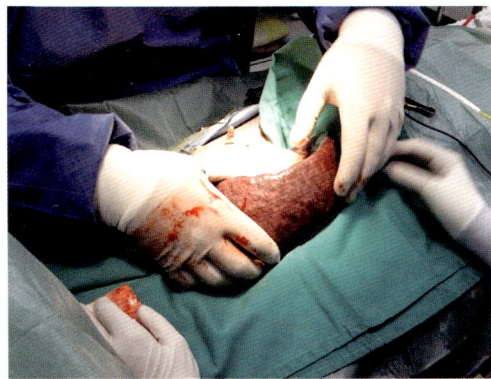

Figure 4. Use of surgical drapes to separate the spleen from the rest of the abdomen prior to splenectomy.

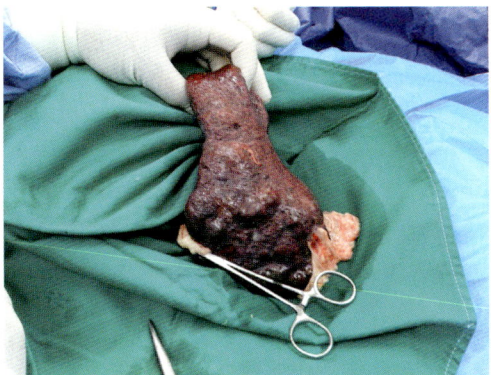

Figure 5. Separation of spleen from the rest of the abdomen.

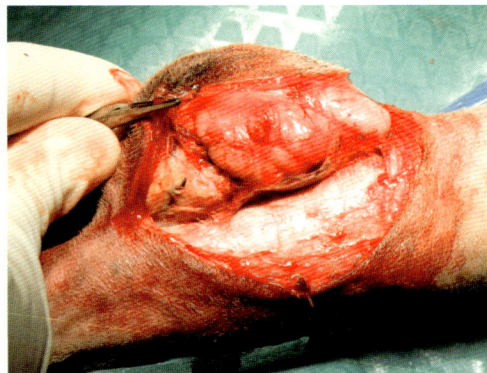

Figure 6. Marginal excision of a soft-tissue sarcoma from a limb. In this case, the surgery was palliative, as the patient had already undergone amputation of another limb.

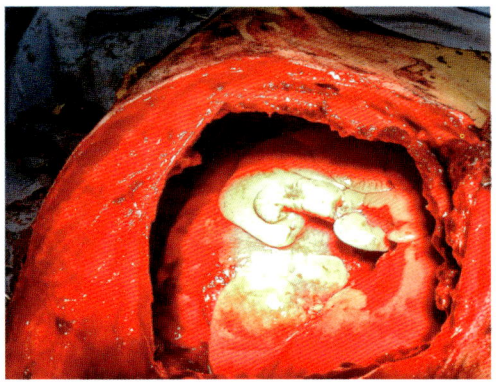

Figure 7. Wide surgical excision of a chondrosarcoma of the rib.

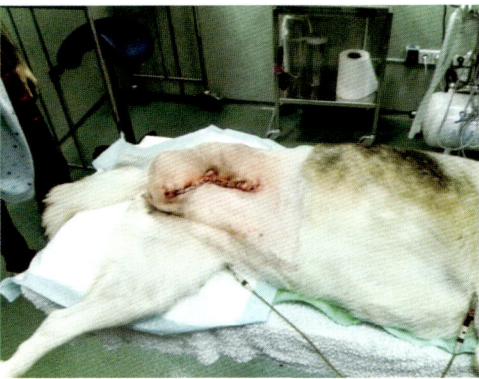

Figure 8. Full amputation of a limb in a patient with tibial osteosarcoma.

> **REGIONAL LYMPH NODES**
>
> Regional lymph node dissection is a controversial topic. On the one hand, sentinel lymph nodes are not always regional and lesions can drain to several lymph node groups (e.g. in the oral cavity). On the other hand, lymphatic drainage may be altered by the presence of a tumour. Removing a healthy lymph node can also be counterproductive. Surgeons must also check that the nodes are not adhered to underlying structures, as capsular rupture can indicate residual disease.

Palliative surgery

The exclusive goal of palliative surgery in cancer is to control local disease. It improves quality of life but has no impact on life expectancy. Pet owners must be clearly informed of the purpose of this type of surgery. A good example of palliative surgery is a splenectomy in an animal with HSA and haemoabdomen.

Types of surgery according to tumour location

- **Thoracic surgery.** Chest cavity tumours include tumours of the lung, mediastinum, heart, trachea, pleura, and chest wall. There are two types of surgery: intercostal thoracotomy for lung or mediastinal tumours and thoracosternotomy for bilateral lung lesions, intrathoracic tracheal lesions, and cranial mediastinal lesions.
- **Abdominal surgery.** This involves an exploratory laparotomy with resection of the mass or excision of the affected organ and exhaustive examination of all other organs, lymph nodes, omentum, and peritoneum to check for disease spread. All suspicious lesions must be biopsied.

Chemotherapy

The cell cycle is divided into four phases (Fig. 9):
- G1. Synthesis of enzymes for DNA replication. This is the phase in which the cell grows. Not all cells reach this phase, remaining instead in the resting G0 phase, where cells do not divide.
- S. Duplication of DNA and associated proteins.
- G2. Synthesis of proteins; beginning of cell division. In this phase, the chromosomes start to condense.
- M. Mitosis.

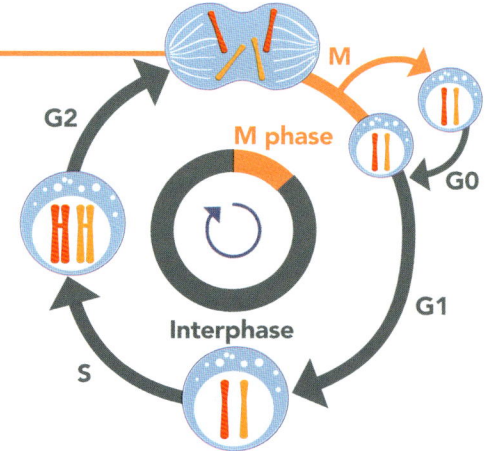

Figure 9. Cell cycle phases.

Neoplasms have a much higher percentage of cells in the cell cycle than healthy tissue. Tumours display a characteristic growth pattern known as a "Gompertz growth curve" (Fig. 10), where the percentage of cells in the cell cycle is highest when the tumour mass cannot yet be detected either radiologically or macroscopically. This is when chemotherapy is most effective.

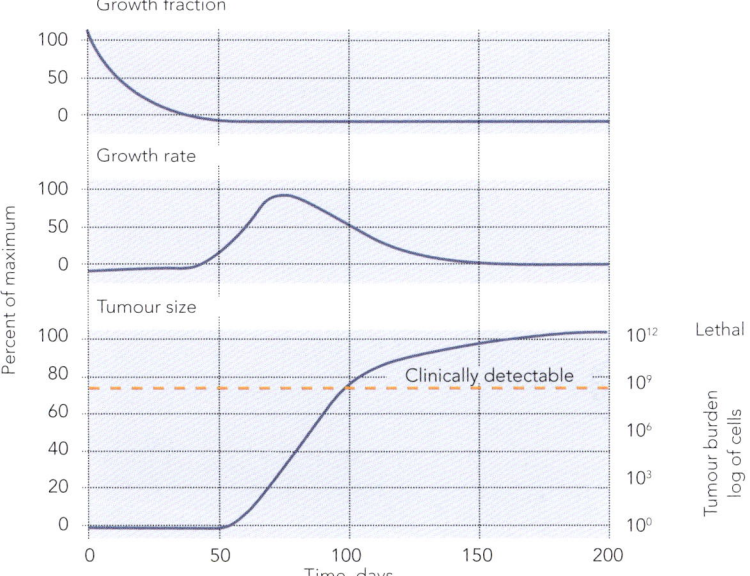

Figure 10.
Gompertz growth curve showing tumour growth.

Chemotherapy refers to the use of cytostatic drugs designed to control tumour growth (preventing recurrences and/or metastases, reducing tumour volume, and inducing tumour remission), while enhancing quality of life and increasing overall survival.

Candidates for chemotherapy are typically geriatric and will therefore have diminished organ reserve capacity (decreased total body water and decreased plasma protein and haemoglobin levels). This should be kept in mind when establishing the dose and frequency of chemotherapy administration. It is also important to monitor hepatic, renal, and cardiac function.

Dosing is normally based on body surface area (m^2), as this correlates best with baseline metabolic activity, blood volume, cardiac output, and pharmacokinetics. In some cases, it is preferable to base calculations on body weight (e.g. when administering doxorubicin to patients weighing <15 kg).

It is important to use and be familiar with the following terms in order to correctly assess response to treatment:
- Complete remission (CR): disappearance of all clinical evidence of a tumour.
- Partial remission (PR): ≥50 % reduction in tumour volume.
- Stable disease (SD): no change.
- Progressive disease (PD): >25 % increase in tumour volume.
- Biological benefit (BB): CR, PR, or SD as long as the patient has an adequate quality of life.

Indications

Generally speaking, chemotherapy is indicated for tumours with known sensitivity to chemotherapy. There are different types and phases of chemotherapy:
- Induction phase: designed to obtain CR.
- Maintenance phase: spacing out of doses to maintain CR/PR, i.e. to maintain SD.
- Rescue phase: administration of new drugs when the tumour enters the PD phase with the aim of achieving CR/PR and restoring SD.
- Adjuvant chemotherapy: administered as complementary treatment (e.g. following a splenectomy in HSA).
- Neoadjuvant chemotherapy: designed to reduce tumour volume and increase the chances of achieving clear margins during subsequent surgery.
- Other modalities: designed to minimise adverse effects and increase treatment effectiveness; examples include intralesional (e.g. in STS), intracavitary, intraperitoneal, intrathoracic, and intrathecal chemotherapy.

The combination of different cytostatic drugs within the same regimen achieves greater control of the neoplasm and also permits the use of lower doses, reducing the likelihood of adverse effects.

Resistance

Resistance is perhaps one of the main limiting factors in chemotherapy. Treatment failure can be due to many resistance mechanisms. Examples are de novo resistance (which occurs in patients undergoing chemotherapy for the first time) and acquired resistance (following a previous course of chemotherapy). Tumours that offer resistance from the outset are probably resistant to all cytostatics.

One strategy for preventing or delaying resistance is to start treatment as early as possible and to use a combination chemotherapy protocol with maximum doses.

Handling of cytostatics

The handling of cytostatics carries health risks related to chronic exposure to small doses. Contamination occurs via the inhalation of airborne particles, skin contact or absorption, or inadvertent ingestion (e.g. when the owner handles the drug in the kitchen). Most cytostatics are mutagenic, teratogenic, or even carcinogenic, and therefore all necessary precautions must be taken.

- **Storage.** The drugs must be clearly labelled, stored in an area with restricted access, and handled only by trained personnel. Most cytostatics must be stored under refrigeration and separated from other drugs.
- **Preparation.** Contamination mostly occurs during drug preparation, but it can be prevented through careful handling in a laminar flow hood and the use of vinyl gloves, a special mask, goggles, and a laboratory coat. In the absence of a laminar flow hood, the following precautions can be taken:
  - Prepare the drug in a quiet, secluded area.
  - Cover the work surface with absorbent paper.
  - Place a filter in the vial.
  - Cover the work surface with gauze soaked in alcohol while reconstituting the solution and filling the syringe.
  - Do not remove the needles from the syringes to prevent contamination by airborne particles and spills.
  - Alternatively, use a closed-system device during drug handling and administration. Closed-system devices consist of applying a double-membrane system to the vial (equipped with an air chamber), syringe, and patient to prevent the release of airborne particles.

Cytostatics in tablet form should not be broken.

- **Administration.** When injecting the drug, use a gauze soaked in alcohol and the same protective clothing as that used for preparing the drug. This step is not necessary when a closed-system device is used.
- **Patient care.** Most cytostatics are strongly irritant (particularly vincristine and doxorubicin) and it is therefore important to ensure that the peripheral venous line is correctly inserted to prevent extravasation. Distressed animals should be sedated. Drugs are eliminated in urine and faeces over a mean period of 48 hours following administration.
- **Disposal.** All utensils used to prepare and administer cytostatic agents must be placed in a plastic bag and disposed of in designated cytotoxic waste containers.

Classification of anticancer drugs

As there is extensive literature on the anticancer drugs available for use in veterinary medicine, this section will focus on those that are most widely used (Fig. 11). The information is presented in table format summarising the main points.

Anticancer drugs are delivered to cancer cells through passive targeting (non-selective targeting that permits the use of higher drug concentrations) or active targeting (a more selective approach that requires a delivery vehicle). Once inside the cells, the drugs act on DNA, enzymes, membranes, and microtubules.

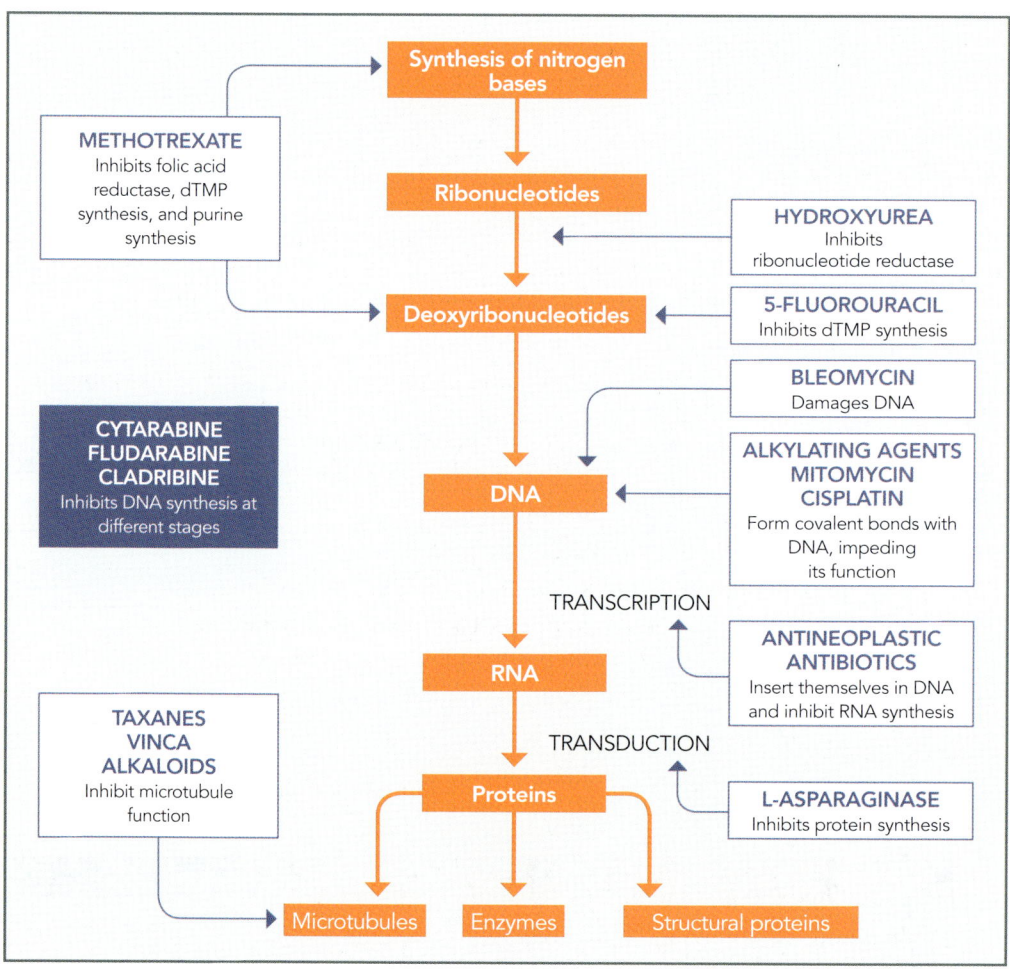

Figure 11. Action of cytostatic drugs at different phases of the cell cycle (from DNA duplication to protein synthesis).

Antibiotics

The toxic and antineoplastic effects of antibiotics are based on the formation of free radicals and the inhibition of topoisomerase II (DNA fragmentation), among other factors.

\multicolumn{2}{c}{Doxorubicin (DXR)}	
Indications	Effective against sarcomas (haemangiosarcoma, osteosarcoma), carcinomas (mammary tumours, squamous cell carcinoma, thyroid cancer), and lymphosarcoma.
Dose	Dogs >15 kg: 30 mg/m² IV for 30 min every 3 wk. Dogs <15 kg and cats: 1 mg/kg/ IV for 30 min every 3 wk. Total maximum dose: 180–240 mg/m².
Administration	Dilute in saline for 40 min. Avoid heparin–saline solutions as heparin can cause the drug to precipitate. Extravasation can result in massive subcutaneous fat and epithelial necrosis. Doxorubicin can cause anaphylactic reactions during administration: • Prevent with methylprednisolone 1–2 mg/kg IV. • Reduce infusion rate if tachycardia, tachypnoea, or hyperthermia is observed (monitor patient). • Perform echocardiography and an electrocardiogram before administration in patients with known heart disease or in patients receiving doses near the maximum total dose.
Storage	Store undiluted at room temperature. 15 days under refrigeration.
Elimination time and route	7 days. Elimination in faeces.
Adverse effects	Vomiting, diarrhoea, colitis, anorexia, pruritus, alopecia, myelosuppression, cardiotoxicity, blisters (vesicant), sepsis, and anaphylaxis.

Mitoxantrone (MTX)	
Indications	Treatment of lymphosarcoma, squamous cell carcinoma, transitional cell carcinoma, mammary tumours, and others. Same indications as for doxorubicin.
Dose and administration	5 mg/m² IV for 5 min every 3 wk.
Storage	Refrigerate once open. 14 days under refrigeration.
Adverse effects	Myelosuppression, thrombocytopaenia, anorexia (cats). Does not produce free radicals (minimally cardiotoxic).

Antimetabolites

Antimetabolites are similar to normal metabolites but they are sufficiently different to interfere with cell multiplication.

5-Fluorouracil	
Indications	Contraindicated in cats (neurological toxicity and death). Treatment of solid and gastrointestinal tumours.
Dose	kg: 5–10 mg/kg IV infusion every wk. m²: 150 mg/m² every wk.
Administration	Intralesional (soft-tissue sarcoma), IV (e.g. canine mammary tumours).
Storage	Room temperature, protected from light.
Elimination time and route	1 day. Eliminated in urine.
Adverse effects	Neurotoxicity (seizures, ataxia), myelosuppression, nausea, gastroenteritis. In cats: death.

Alkylating agents

Alkylating agents cause DNA modifications that prevent normal DNA activity.

Cyclophosphamide (CPX)	
Indications	One of the most widely used cytostatics in veterinary medicine. Leukaemia, lymphosarcoma, soft-tissue sarcoma, and mammary tumours. Metronomic therapy.
Dose and administration	PO: 50 mg/m² for 4 consecutive days every 3 wk. IV: 200 mg/m² infusion with saline for 20 min every 3 wk. Per protocol.
Elimination time and route	3 days. Mainly in urine.
Storage	Room temperature. Once reconstituted: 24 hours at room temperature; 6 days under refrigeration.
Preparation	Water for injection.
Adverse effects	Myelosuppression, neurotoxicity, gastroenteritis, and sterile haemorrhagic cystitis, which is prevented by forcing diuresis with furosemide on the morning of administration to favour bladder emptying (this prevents contact between the metabolite acrolein and the bladder wall).

Chlorambucil	
Indications	Tends to be used instead of cyclophosphamide when this is not tolerated. Leukaemia, chronic lymphocytic leukaemia, and mast cell tumours.
Dose	kg: 0.1 mg/kg every 24–48 h. m²: 2–8 mg/m² every 24–48 h. 20 mg/m² every 2 wk. Metronomic therapy.
Administration	Oral.
Elimination time and route	1 day. Eliminated in urine.
Storage	Room temperature/refrigeration.
Adverse effects	Myelosuppression, gastroenteritis.

Lomustine (CCNU)	
Indications	Nervous system tumours, lymphosarcoma, and mast cell tumours.
Dose and administration	Dogs: 70–90 mg/m² PO every 3 wk. Cats: 50 mg/m² PO every 5–6 wk.
Storage	Room temperature.
Elimination time and route	1 day. Metabolised in the liver and kidneys.
Adverse effects	Myelosuppression, accumulative thrombocytopaenia (after 1–4 weeks of treatment), liver failure, pulmonary insufficiency, gastroenteritis.

Vinca alkaloids

Vinca alkaloids inhibit the synthesis of tubulin and/or the microtubules necessary for cell division.

Vincristine (VC)	
Indications	Widely used in veterinary medicine (very well tolerated by cats); used in many protocols. Normally combined with cyclophosphamide and prednisone.
Dose and administration	0.5–0.75 mg/m² IV.
Storage	28 days under refrigeration. Saline preparation.
Elimination time and route	7 days. Urine and faeces.
Adverse effects	Myelosuppression, neurotoxicity with paresthesia, blistering, ileus.

Vinblastine (VB)	
Indications	Can be used instead of vincristine with some limitations. Treatment of mast cell tumours, lymphosarcoma.
Dose and administration	2 mg/m² IV bolus every 1–2 wk. Preferably diluted in saline.
Storage	Under refrigeration once reconstituted; stable for 30 days.
Elimination time and route	3 days. Eliminated in urine.
Adverse effects	Myelosuppression, gastrointestinal irritation, neurotoxicity, and mild peripheral neuropathy (less serious than with vincristine), blistering.

Platinum-based agents

Platinum-based agents form complexes that bind to DNA, inhibiting its activity.

Cisplatin	
Indications	Inoperable or disseminated carcinomas. Contraindicated in cats: respiratory toxicity with hydrothorax and pulmonary and mediastinal oedema that are generally fatal.
Dose and administration	60–70 mg/m² IV for 30 min every 3 wk; infusion with saline to prevent neurotoxicity and acute kidney failure. Tends to be administered in isolation either intravenously or intralesionally. Insert a catheter and administer: • Saline for 6 hours. • Cisplatin for 4 hours (total dose diluted in saline). • Saline for another 4 hours. • Force and monitor diuresis via a urinary probe.
Storage	Protect from light. Freeze once reconstituted (3 weeks).
Elimination time and route	1 day. Eliminated in urine.
Adverse effects	Dose-dependent vomiting during administration that can be prevented by maropitant, butorphanol, or ondansetron. Avoid contact with aluminium and aluminium derivatives. Neurotoxicity, gastroenteritis, myelosuppression, acute kidney injury, hearing loss.

Carboplatin	
Indications	Cisplatin analogue not associated with nephrotoxicity.
	Can be used in cats.
Preparation	Avoid contact with aluminium.
	Dilute in water for IV injection.
Dose and administration	300 mg/m² IV 20 min every 3 wk.
	Dilute in dextrose 5 %; intravenous or intralesional/intracavitary administration.
Storage	Protect from light.
	Remains stable for 8 hours after reconstitution.
Elimination time and route	1 day. Eliminated in urine.
Adverse effects	Myelosuppression, gastroenteritis, allergic reactions.

Other

Corticosteroids (cause DNA fragmentation in sensitive cells)	
Indications	Useful for managing hypercalcaemia and controlling pain, intracranial pressure, and hypoglycaemia.
Dose and administration (prednisone)	kg: 1 mg/kg/d every 4 wk, 1 mg/kg/48 h until tumour remission.
	m²: 30–40 mg/m²/d.

NSAIDs
See next.

Adverse effects of chemotherapy

The cytotoxic effects of chemotherapy are dose-dependent in both normal and neoplastic cells as both populations undergo the same cell cycle phases. The populations most frequently affected are bone marrow cells, gastrointestinal epithelial cells, and to a lesser extent, hair follicle cells.

The vast majority of cytostatic drugs only act in one of these phases.

Because of the toxicity of these drugs, the narrow dose range possible, and the advanced age of many of the patients, owners must be properly informed about potential adverse effects, about how to prevent and treat them, and about when they should bring their pet to the emergency department.

All cytostatics reach their nadir about 7–12 days after administration. In some cases (lomustine, carboplatin), thrombocytopaenia can occur after several doses. In such cases, the drug must be withdrawn due to the risk of spontaneous bleeding.

The most common adverse effects of chemotherapy are described next.

Iatrogenic Cushing's disease
- Caused by the long-term use of corticosteroids (in lymphosarcoma [LSA], MCT).
- Dogs are much more sensitive than cats.
- Long-term effects include leukopaenia and thrombocytopaenia.

Bone marrow toxicity
Bone marrow toxicity is relatively common due to the high proliferative activity of bone marrow cells. A total white blood cell (WBC) count should be performed before all chemotherapy sessions. A **neutrophil count** is also desirable, as is manual confirmation of the WBC differential on a blood smear.

Suppression is greatest in geriatric patients due to the bone marrow's reduced functionality and ability to recover. Red blood cell counts can be affected by long-term treatment.

Neutropaenia
Neutropaenia is the most serious adverse effect of chemotherapy. The protocol for action in such cases is shown in Table 1.

Table 1. Protocol for action following detection of chemotherapy-induced neutropaenia.

Total neutrophil count	Fever	Clinical signs	Treatment
<3000/µl	No	No	Delay the next dose. Do not administer antibiotics.
	Yes	No	Delay the next dose. Antibiotics and close outpatient follow-up.
<1500/µl	No	No	Delay the next dose. Prophylactic antibiotics on an outpatient basis.
	Yes	Yes	Delay the next dose. Hospitalisation and close monitoring due to risk of sepsis. IV antibiotics: • Trimethoprim–sulfamethoxazole 15 mg/kg/12 h. • Cephalexin 22 mg/kg/12 h. • Cefoxitin 22 mg/kg/12 h. • Ampicillin 22 mg/kg/12 h. • Amoxicillin and clavulanic acid 22 mg/kg/4–6–8 h. • Enrofloxacin 5–10 mg/kg/12–24 h.

Adapted from *BSVA Manual of Canine and Feline Oncology* (2004).

Neutropaenia is the main limiting factor in chemotherapy. Sufficient time should be taken to explain the consequences of this complication to owners. These, in turn, should be instructed to take their pet's rectal temperature at home and to administer prophylactic antibiotics (trimethoprim–sulfamethoxazole) if this reaches 39–39.5 °C. If a higher temperature is detected, the pet should be brought it for emergency care as temperatures >39.5 °C are associated with a risk of sepsis due to bacterial translocation (enterohepatic circulation).

Other signs of neutropaenia are lethargy, weakness, and poor general health. Patients with sepsis should be administered both intravenous fluids (to treat shock and restore electrolytes) and intravenous broad-spectrum antibiotics (amoxicillin and clavulanic acid with or without quinolones and/or metronidazole). Blood, urine, and bronchial aspirate cultures are also recommended. Finally, the need for a full blood transfusion should be evaluated.

Thrombocytopaenia
- Typically seen in patients treated with platinum-based drugs and lomustine.
- Normally asymptomatic until it drops to a level at which it can cause spontaneous bleeding.
- Proposed limit for interrupting treatment: <60,000 μl.

Anaemia
- Occurs after long treatment periods (haematocrit values <20 %).
- Paraneoplastic syndromes must be ruled out.
- Clinical signs: weakness, anorexia, tachycardia, and tachypnoea.
- Can generally be resolved by reducing treatment dose or increasing interval between doses.

Organ sensitivity
Myelosuppression. Seen with the vast majority of cytostatics.
Gastrointestinal alterations. The most common gastrointestinal effects are nausea, vomiting, diarrhoea, and colitis. Corticosteroids and nonsteroidal anti-inflammatory drugs (NSAIDs) can cause ulcers and bleeding and interfere with gastric mucosal protection. Symptomatic treatment must be administered and infection by *Giardia*, *Clostridium*, or other parasites ruled out.
Cardiotoxicity. The cumulative effect of doxorubicin can cause dilated cardiomyopathies and transient arrhythmias in predisposed breeds and in animals with pre-existing heart disease. The maximum tolerated dose established for dogs is 180–240 mg/m^2 (over 6–8 sessions).
Lung parenchyma. Caused by treatment with cisplatin (lethal in cats).
Hepatotoxicity. Caused by treatment with NSAIDs, corticosteroids, and lomustine.
Kidney alterations. Caused by treatment with cisplatin or doxorubicin (in cats). They can be prevented by avoiding these drugs in patients with known kidney disease. An appropriate fluid therapy and diuresis protocol should be implemented for patients with adequate kidney function.
Bladder alterations. Seen in patients treated with cyclophosphamide. Metabolism of this drug in the liver produces metabolites that have an irritant effect on the bladder mucosa. The resulting irritation varies according to the time that the metabolite acrolein is in contact with the mucosa. It can generally be avoided by

previous administration of furosemide 1–2 mg/kg and, where possible, administration of cyclophosphamide in the morning. Cystitis should be treated symptomatically (with NSAIDs in patients with adequate kidney function), and antibiotics should be administered for secondary infections.

Neurological disorders. Caused by vinca alkaloids (neuropathies), cisplatin (hearing loss), and 5-fluorouracil (seizures, lethal in cats).

Eye complications. Caused by cisplatin (blindness).

Hypersensitivity reactions. Caused by doxorubicin (erythema, trembling, or vomiting). These can generally be controlled by reducing the infusion rate and premedicating with maropitant, corticosteroids, or diphenhydramine.

Special considerations

Cisplatin. Never use in cats. Avoid in patients with impaired kidney function.

Doxorubicin. Use with caution in patients with known heart disease or in predisposed breeds (Dobermans, Boxers). Use with caution in animals with kidney disease. Doxorubicin has high vesicant potential.

Vesicants and extravasation. Most cytostatic drugs are irritant to a greater or lesser degree. The effects of extravasation tend to manifest as blistering or severe erythema at the injection site. Constant licking is a common observation as the sores are generally very painful.

Vesicant potential is high for doxorubicin, moderate for vincristine, and mild/moderate for cisplatin, methotrexate, and 5-flourouracil.

Blistering and necrosis advance very fast, and the extent of tissue damage is proportional to the amount of extravasated drug. When extravasation occurs, it is important to stop administration of the drug immediately and draw 5–10 ml of blood (and any traces of the extravasated drug) from the surrounding subcutaneous tissue before removing the catheter. The specific steps required to treat extravasation vary according to the drug used:

- Doxorubicin
    - Apply cold compresses (vasoconstriction).
    - Administer dexrazoxane IV at a dose 10 times that of doxorubicin for 3 hours following extravasation. Repeat at 24 and 48 hours.
    - Apply topical dimethyl sulphoxide (DMSO) every 2–4 hours.
    - Apply an anti-inflammatory corticosteroid ointment.
- Vincristine
    - Apply hot compresses.
    - Inject 1500 units of hyaluronidase.
    - Apply an anti-inflammatory corticosteroid ointment.

In the case of both doxorubicin and vincristine, lesions tend to appear within 3–10 days of administering the drug. If the reaction is confined and detected in time, **wide surgical excision** of the necrotic tissue can be contemplated. If damage is extensive, the affected limb will need to be amputated.

Radiation therapy

Principles of radiobiology

Ionising radiation causes chemical changes in live material (and DNA in particular) through cleavage of covalent bonds and formation of free radicals. The changes occur either directly (through absorption of radiation by DNA) or indirectly (through absorption of radiation by water, resulting in the formation of free radicals that react with and damage DNA [radiolysis]). Radiation can cause base-pair deletion, cleavage of hydrogen bonds, single- or double-strand DNA breaks, and locally multiply damage sites (LMDS).

Highly proliferative cells are more sensitive to ionising radiation. Certain epithelial tissues are particularly sensitive to the effects of radiation (**early-response tissue**). Tissues with a lower proliferation rate are known as **late-response tissues**.

Put very simply, a certain amount of damage is "absorbed" by early-response tissue in each session. Late-response tissue, by contrast, is damaged by cumulative exposure over the course of treatment.

The goal of radiation therapy is to destroy as many tumour cells as possible while minimising the impact on healthy tissue. This is achieved through dose fractionation, which consists of administering the total dose in several treatment sessions over a given period. Careful management of variables such as total dose, number of sessions (fractionation), and time is an essential part of protocol design.

Radiation is measured in Gray (Gy) (1 joule/kg or 100 rad).

Fractionation is important as tumour cells and early- and late-response tissues have different repair capabilities. The use of small doses of radiation results in the survival of a higher proportion of late-response tissue cells than tumour cells.

Cell redistribution refers to the fact that cells in different phases of the cell cycle display different sensitivity to radiation. M- and G2-phase cells, for example, are more sensitive than S- or G1-phase cells. After a radiation session, cells in the "radioresistant" phase move into the sensitive phases.

The presence of hypoxic tumour areas also reduces the effectiveness of radiation therapy. However, in the interval between radiation fractions, tumours become more aerobic (reoxygenation) and therefore more radiosensitive.

Cell repopulation occurs in both tumours and early-response tissues (mucosa, skin), and therefore the goal of radiation therapy is to administer a dose that minimises the repopulation of tumours but allows the recovery of healthy, early-response tissue. In the case of late-response tissue, dose per fraction is more important than the duration of treatment.

While hyperfractionated protocols (5 days a week for 5–8 weeks) are used in human medicine, veterinary protocols typically use 3–4 sessions a week (Monday, Wednesday, and Friday) because of geographic limitations and the need for anaesthesia. Thanks to advances in anaesthetic techniques, it is now possible to schedule two sessions a day in certain cases. These sessions must be separated by at least 6 hours, which is the estimated time it takes for DNA repair to occur in healthy tissue.

The total dose used in any protocol should be calculated to minimise the risk of late reactions in healthy tissue in the irradiated area. The theoretical benefits of protocols that use small doses per fraction seem to be evident, as they allow a higher total dose to be administered without increasing the risk of late effects. Excessive treatment duration, by contrast, permits tumour repopulation, which can negatively affect disease control.

The total dose tolerated also depends on other factors, such as the type of healthy late-response tissue in the irradiated area (the brain and spinal cord are more sensitive than muscle or bone) and the volume of tissue to irradiate (large volumes of healthy tissue are more sensitive).

Equipment

Ionising radiation can be applied through an external source (external beam radiation therapy) or through radioactive isotopes (brachytherapy). External beam radiation therapy is the most widely used system in veterinary medicine. Orthovoltage radiation operates with voltages in the range of 150–500 hVp. This is the oldest system and is now practically in disuse. Megavoltage radiation operates with mean voltages >1000 electron volts (MeV), which permits excellent tissue penetration. It is applied using machines with a radioactive source (cobalt pump) or linear accelerators, which generate high-energy photons (Fig. 12).

Some linear accelerators can emit electrons as well as photons as a source of radiation. Electrons have a limited penetration capacity and are an interesting option for irradiating superficial tumours, as the underlying structures are spared (Fig. 13).

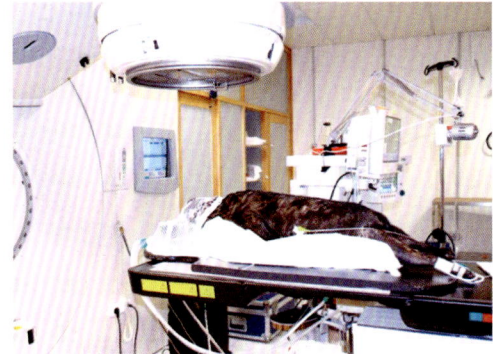
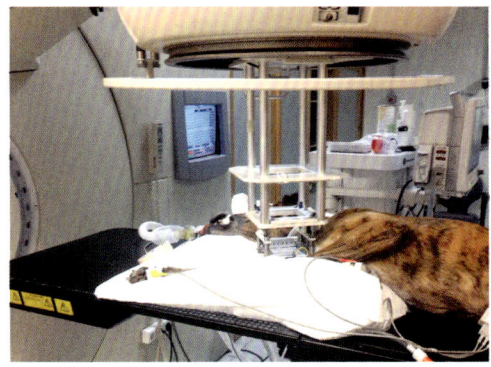

Figure 12. Linear accelerator, treatment with photons.

Figure 13. Linear accelerator, treatment with electrons.

Computerised radiation therapy planning systems can be used to combine photon beams from different angles while applying a minimum dose to healthy adjacent tissue.
- **Three-dimensional conformal therapy radiation therapy (3DCRT)** allows for better adaptation of the irradiated field to the geometric shape of the tumour. It requires the importing of images (normally computed tomography images) into the planning system and the use of fixation systems that reproduce the exact position of the animal in each treatment session. Examples of positioning systems are vacuum bags, resin moulds, and thermoplastic masks. It is not uncommon for several of these systems to be used simultaneously (Fig. 14).

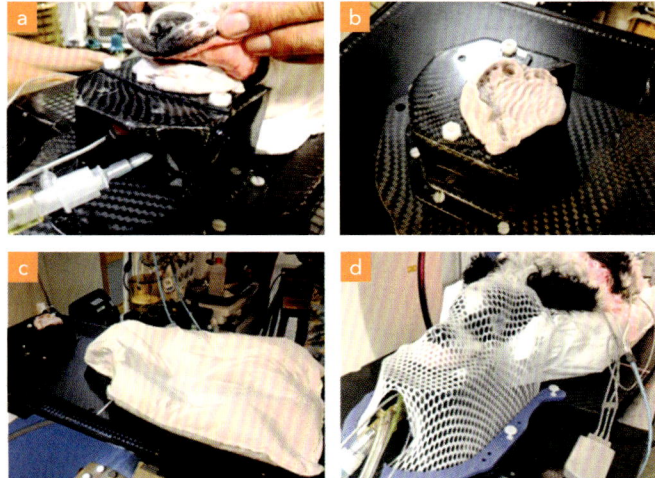

Figure 14. Positioning systems Resin mould (a and b). Vacuum bag (c). Thermoplastic mask (d).

- **Intensity-modulated radiation therapy (IMRT)** is an advanced form of 3DCRT that is delivered by a computer-controlled multileaf collimator that allows more accurate 3-dimensional dose administration through the modulation of photon beam intensity. It also permits the use of higher doses in the treatment area by minimising the dose absorbed by healthy tissue. It is particularly useful in the treatment of tumours of the head and neck as it spares damage to structures such as the eyes and brain (Fig. 15).

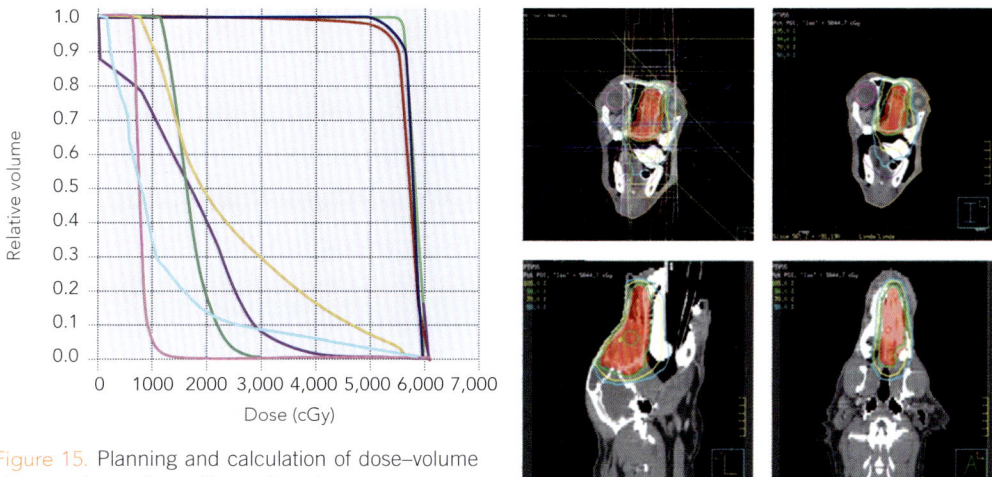

Figure 15. Planning and calculation of dose–volume histogram in a patient with nasal carcinoma.

Indications

As a general rule, radiation therapy is indicated for localised solid tumours in patients with residual disease or in which surgical excision is contraindicated.
- **Nasal cavity tumours.** Best option for nasal cavity tumours and generally associated with a survival time >400 days.
- **Oral cavity tumours.** Helps to achieve local control when administered as monotherapy or adjuvant therapy.
- **Tumours of the central nervous system.** Associated with survival times of almost 2 years depending on the type of tumour. Achieves complete or partial resolution of endocrine-related disorders in patients with pituitary tumours (Fig. 16).
- **Cutaneous carcinoma, soft tissue sarcoma, and mast cell tumours.** Lengthens disease-free time in patients that undergo surgical excision without margins.
- **Bone tumours.** Highly effective pain-control strategy when amputation is not an option (orthopaedic reasons or rejection by owner).
- **Lymphosarcoma.** Used for stage I or localised mucocutaneous lymphomas.

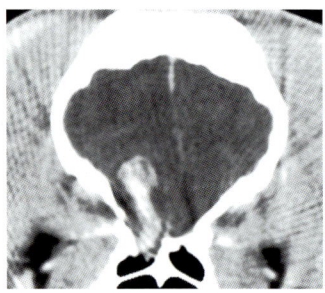 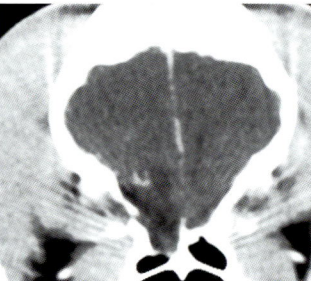

Figure 16. CT scans of an intracranial tumour before and after treatment.

Adverse effects

Radiation-induced adverse effects are classified as late or acute.

Late effects occur in slowly proliferating tissue (bone, lung, heart, kidney, or spinal cord) and can be severe (fibrosis, necrosis, or loss of function) and sometimes difficult to manage. The radiation dose is limited by tolerance of the healthy tissue within the radiation field.

Acute adverse effects involve highly proliferating tissue (oral mucosa, intestinal epithelium, eyes, or skin) and occur shortly after treatment initiation. They are generally self-limiting and resolve within 2–3 weeks.

Mucositis refers to inflammation of the mucosa of the oral cavity, pharynx, and/or oesophagus as a result of radiation to the head or neck. It always occurs, albeit with varying degrees of severity, during the treatment of oral tumours. It typically appears during the second week of treatment. Common signs are oral sensitivity or thick saliva, which can cause patients to reject food or water. In such cases, they should be fed a soft, tasty diet low in salt. Mucositis resolves 2–3 weeks after treatment ends. It can also occur during treatment of any portion of the digestive tract (e.g. radiation of the bladder tends to produce colitis).

Radiodermatitis is an acute dose-dependent reaction that affects the treatment area and has highly variable manifestations. Alopecia is common and can be permanent or take months to resolve. Damage to melanocytes can cause both depigmentation and hyperpigmentation. Hair loss tends to be accompanied by dry desquamation. Wet desquamation can occur between the third and fifth week of treatment initiation and causes pruritus or pain and even secondary infections. It is important to keep the treated area clean and uncovered and to use desiccating antiseptics (chlorhexidine) and, where indicated, corticosteroids and/or antibiotics.

Eyes are highly sensitive to radiation and the adverse effects are dose-dependent. Acute effects include blepharitis, blepharospasm, conjunctivitis, and temporary or permanent dry keratoconjunctivitis. Late effects include vascular alterations and cataracts.

Antiangiogenic therapy

New treatment options such as metronomic therapy have appeared in recent years, opening up new possibilities, particularly for elderly patients and patients that do not respond to other treatments. Nonetheless, owners must be adequately informed, as the effectiveness of metronomic therapy has not been demonstrated to date.

Metronomic therapy involves the administration of low doses every 24–48 hours over long periods of time.

Angiogenesis is continually activated as a tumour progresses, favouring further growth, invasive capacity, and metastatic potential. For a tumour to grow between 3–4 mm it needs to be "fed" by newly formed blood vessels. Inhibiting angiogenesis should therefore help to control tumour development.

Metronomic therapy has evident advantages: it is less toxic, more affordable, and, in some cases, appears to increase life expectancy.

In addition, it is capable of modifying the tumour microenvironment without exerting significant cytotoxic effects. One of the main modifications is inhibition of angiogenesis:
- Endothelial blood vessel cells in tumours are much more sensitive than healthy tissue cells to cytostatic drugs.
- Metronomic therapy targets progenitor endothelial cells, which are produced by the bone marrow and transported to the tumour through the bloodstream. With conventional chemotherapy, these cells increase in number during rest periods.
- Metronomic therapy acts on different proangiogenic and antiangiogenic factors.
- It is thought to reduce the number of T regulatory cells (Tregs) that inhibit cell immunity and stimulate dendritic cells.

Few studies have analysed the safety and efficacy of metronomic therapy in veterinary medicine (STS with incomplete excision, stage II splenic HSA, transitional cell carcinoma [chlorambucil], and different tumours that have proven refractory to conventional treatments). The results of these studies suggest that this modality has a stabilising effect on the tumour, which, in itself, constitutes a considerable clinical benefit for the patient.

Several studies have analysed the use of cyclophosphamide (12.5–25 mg/m² every 24–48 h), chlorambucil, and lomustine used in isolation or combined with different NSAIDs. Few adverse effects (occasional haemorrhagic cystitis) have been reported to date.

Metronomic therapy administered either during or after conventional therapy is gradually emerging as an alternative for tumours that are refractory to other treatments.

Most protocols combine a cytostatic drug and an NSAID, although drugs such as thalidomide and pioglitazone are sometimes used.

The most widely used cytostatics are cyclophosphamide 10–15 mg/m² every 24–48 h and chlorambucil 2–4 mg/m² every 24–48 h.

Tyrosine kinase inhibitors

Biology

Protein kinases are key molecules in the regulation of intracellular signals. They regulate processes related to cell survival, division, migration, and differentiation. Kinases act via the phosphorylation of other proteins. They use ATP as a source of phosphate, which can result in the binding of an amino acid to another protein or to itself, leading to a conformational change and triggering a cascade signal. This occurs in response to a stimulus triggered by a growth factor or another extracellular substance.

Protein kinases are known as tyrosine kinases (TKs) when they phosphorylate proteins at a tyrosine amino acid and as serine–threonine kinases when they phosphorylate serine–threonine residues. Tyrosine kinases are located in cell membranes, cytoplasms, and nuclei (Fig. 17).

Their receptors (TKRs) are cell membrane TKs that are stimulated by growth factors and cytokines, among other factors, These receptors have an extracellular domain, a transmembrane domain, and an intracytoplasmic domain, which is where phosphorylation occurs.

Some TKRs have a very important role in processes such as angiogenesis. Examples are vascular endothelial growth factor receptor (VEGFR), platelet-derived growth factor receptor (PDGFR), fibroblast growth factor receptor (FGFR), and angiopoietin receptors (Tie-1 and Tie-2). VEGFR is located in immature blood vessels and its activation induces the proliferation and migration of endothelial cells, while PDGFR is located in pericytes and is involved in their proliferation. FGFR, in turn, is found in endothelial cells and its stimulation increases the expression of VEGF. Both Tie-1 and Tie-2 are found in tumour blood vessels and have an important role in the recruitment of pericytes and smooth muscle cells for the new vascular bed.

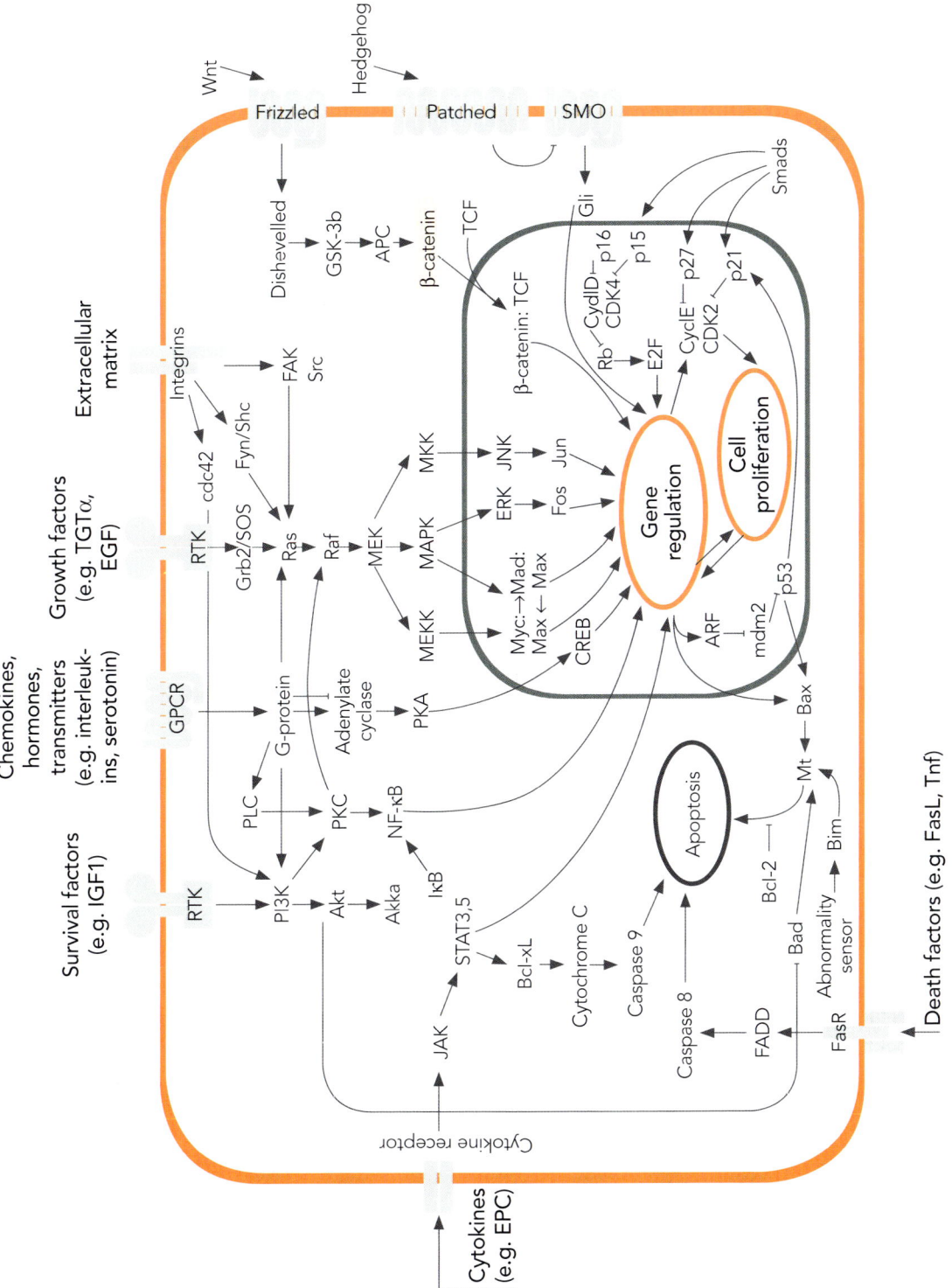

Figure 17. Main intracellular signalling pathways. Adapted from https://en.wikipedia.org/wiki/File:Signal_transduction_v1.png. By Roadnottaken at the English language Wikipedia, CC BY-SA 3.0, https://commons.wikimedia.org/w/index.php?curid=2163484.

Cytoplasmic TKs act by transmitting signals generated by TKRs to the nucleus through intermediaries that are also phosphorylated. There are two cytoplasmic signalling pathways that are often dysregulated in tumour cells.
- The first is the RAS-RAF-MEK-ERK/p38/JNK pathway (which controls the cell cycle). Some components of this pathway (e.g. RAS) are frequently mutated in numerous tumours.
- The second pathway (phosphatidyl inositol-3-kinase) phosphorylates AKT, which, in turn, activates different proteins involved in cell cycle regulation, cell survival (inhibition of apoptosis), and cell growth.

Once the signal crosses the cytoplasm and enters the nucleus, it alters gene transcription and proteins that regulate the cell cycle.

Table 2. Kinase mutations in tumour cells described in human medicine.

Tyrosine kinase	Associated cancer
EGFR family	Mammary, ovarian, lung, stomach, colon, glioblastomas.
Insulin receptor family	Sarcomas, cervical and renal cancer.
PDGFR family	Glioblastomas, ovarian cancer, chronic myeloid leukaemia.
KIT	Acute myeloid leukaemia, gastrointestinal stromal tumour, seminoma, mast cell tumour, lung cancer.
Flt3	Acute myeloid leukaemia.
VEGFR family	Angiogenesis, Kaposi sarcoma, haemangiosarcoma, melanoma.
FGFR family	Acute myeloid leukaemia, lymphoma, prostate and mammary cancer, multiple myeloma.
NGFR family	Thyroid cancer, neuroblastoma, fibrosarcoma, acute myeloid leukaemia.
Met/Ron	Thyroid cancer, osteosarcoma, rhabdomyosarcoma, liver, kidney, and colon cancer.
EPHR family	Melanoma, stomach, colon, mammary, and oesophageal cancer.
AXL	Acute myeloid leukaemia.
Tie family	Angiogenesis, stomach cancer, haemangioblastoma.
RET family	Thyroid cancer, multiple endocrine neoplastic syndrome.
ALK	Non-Hodgkin lymphoma.

Kinase inhibition

Tyrosine kinase dysregulation due to mutations (Table 2), overexpression, or chromosomal translocation can result in the permanent activation of cell proliferation or survival mechanisms or apoptosis-inhibition mechanisms.

Approximately 40 % of dogs suffering from MCT have a mutation in the KIT receptor (a TKR) that causes permanent activation of this receptor (in the absence of its growth factor), resulting in uncontrolled cell proliferation and increased survival. A similar situation has been described for B-raf kinase in canine transitional cell carcinoma (TCC) of the bladder; mutations of the *BRAF* gene have been detected in 80 % of cases.

Discovery of mutations such as these has led to the growing use of **targeted therapies**, whose aim is to block these molecules through monoclonal antibodies (not yet available for veterinary use) or small inhibitory molecules. Inhibitory molecules act by blocking the kinase ATP binding site (competitive inhibitors) or the interaction between proteins (allosteric or noncompetitive inhibition).

Tyrosine kinase inhibitors in veterinary medicine

Two TK inhibitors have been described to date in the treatment of canine MCT.

Toceranib phosphate

Toceranib phosphate is an orally bioavailable inhibitor that blocks several TKRs, such as VEGFR2, PDGFRα, and KIT.

The maximum tolerated dose, established at 3.25 mg/kg every 48 h, was associated with several adverse effects (mostly gastrointestinal). A lower dose of 2.4 mg/kg exerted a similar biological effect but was better tolerated.

Toceranib has been used to treat many solid tumours, and has been found to be biologically active against apocrine gland adenocarcinoma of the anal sac, metastatic osteosarcoma, thyroid carcinoma, nasal carcinoma, and head and neck carcinoma (Fig. 18).

Administration of toceranib and an NSAID on alternate days has been proposed as a strategy for minimising gastrointestinal effects.

One study from 2013 showed that toceranib (2.5 mg/kg toceranib on Monday–Wednesday–Friday) combined with cytotoxic drugs at metronomic doses and cyclooxygenase (COX) 2 inhibitors achieved an objective clinical response.

Researchers who have started to investigate the combination of toceranib and conventional chemotherapy (toceranib with vinblastine for the treatment of MCTs, toceranib with lomustine, etc.) have found neutropaenia to be the main limiting factor.

The combination of toceranib and radiation therapy (6 Gy once a week for 4 weeks) resulted in a response rate of 76.4 % and a complete response rate of 58.8 % in inoperable MCTs.

The first prospective study of toceranib in cats with different types of tumours was published in 2013. The study analysed 21 animals administered a mean dose of 2.8 mg/kg on Monday–Wednesday–Friday. Most of the cats tolerated the treatment and the clinical response rate was 21 %.

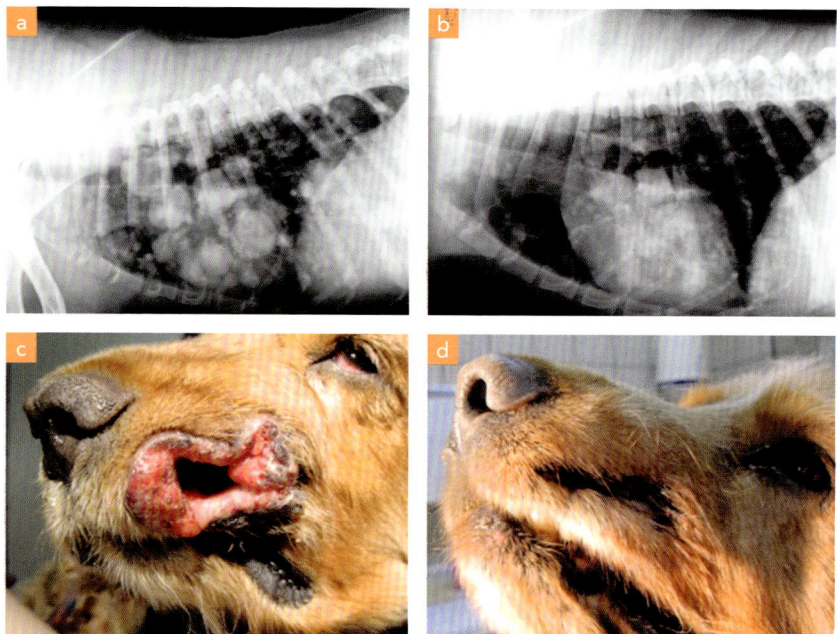

Figure 18. Clinical responses to treatment with toceranib. Dog with metastasis from thyroid cancer before treatment with toceranib and an NSAID (a) and clinical response at 30 days (b). Dog with squamous cell carcinoma before treatment with toceranib (c) and response to treatment (d). *Images courtesy of Elena Martínez de Merlo.*

Masitinib

Masitinib is a TK inhibitor that blocks the KIT receptor, PDGFRα/β, and the cytoplasmic kinase Lyn. It is administered at a dose of 12.5 mg/kg every 24 h.

In a recent study of 10 dogs with epitheliotropic cutaneous lymphoma, masitinib achieved two complete responses and five partial responses.

A 50-mg dose of masitinib every 48 hours has been shown to be safe in healthy cats, which opens the door for the use of this inhibitor in feline tumours with KIT or PDGFR overexpression or mutations.

Immunotherapy

The main function of the immune system is to protect against infectious agents, although its ability to rearrange and eliminate neoplastic cells is also key in cancer biology. The immune system is designed to recognise aberrant proteins, such those altered during carcinogenesis. These proteins are known as tumour antigens.

Evidence that the immune system has an antitumour role includes remissions in untreated patients, detection of Tregs and monocytic, lymphocytic, and plasmocytic infiltrates, occurrence of certain neoplasms in immunodepressed animals, and reports of tumour remission induced by immunomodulatory agents.

Immunity can be innate or acquired. **The innate immune system** is a fast-acting system with low specificity formed by natural physiological barriers (skin and mucosa), complement proteins, phagocytes (macrophages, neutrophils, natural killer cells, and dendritic cells), and cytokines, which regulate and coordinate the different cells involved in the innate immune defence system. **The acquired immune system** allows the organism to "remember" pathogenic agents with which it has had previous contact, and accordingly to distinguish between innate and external components. It is composed of B cells (CD79$^+$) and T cells (CD3$^+$). Depending on their CD (cluster of differentiation) or MHC (major histocompatibility complex) molecules, T cells (cell-mediated immune response) are classified as **cytoxic T cells (Tc, CD3, CD8, class I MHC) or T helper cells** (Th, CD3, CD4, class II MHC), which are further divided into Th1 and Th2 cells. There are also Tregs and natural killer cells. B cells synthesise antibodies (humoral system) that activate the complement cascade, increase phagocytic capacity, and induce antibody-dependent cytotoxicity.

The term "cancer immunosurveillance" refers to the idea that the immune system can prevent cancer from developing.

A tumour can evade the immune system through several mechanisms:
- Presence of myeloid-derived suppressor cells (MDSCs) and tumour-associated macrophages (TAMs). There is a correlation between the presence of these cells and both clinical stage and the presence of metastasis in solid tumours.
- Increase in the immunosuppressive cell population (Tregs).
- Presence of immunosuppressive cytokines (interleukin 10 [IL-10]).
- Inactivation or alteration of dendritic cell maturation.
- Loss of MHC class I molecules.
- Reduced expression of B7-1, a protein that mediates T-cell adhesion to MHC class I molecules.

Biological response modifiers

Biological response modifiers (BRMs) are molecules that can modify naturally occurring responses to changes in the microenvironment. Examples are oncolytic viruses, which are used in human and veterinary medicine. Both in vitro and in vivo tests have shown that these viruses effectively infect target tumour cells without causing major adverse effects. Work on oncolytic virus therapy is ongoing.

Another novel BRM is the toll-like receptor 7 (TLR-7) agonist imiquimod, which has shown successful results in patients with Bowen's disease (multicentric carcinoma and in situ SCC). TLR-7 forms part of the innate immune response and is found on the surface of macrophages and dendritic cells. One study reported response in all 12 cats with Bowen's disease treated with topical 5 % imiquimod cream.

Recombinant cytokines

Several studies have described the use of recombinant cytokines in human and veterinary medicine. One example is feline interleukin-2 (vCP1338), which is designed to reduce the risk of recurrence in cats with ISS. It is used as an adjuvant to surgery and radiation therapy.

Antitumour vaccines

The ultimate goal of antitumour vaccines is to trigger an antitumour immune response that results in the clinical regression of tumours and metastases. Various vaccines are currently being developed for different tumours.

One example, not yet available in all countries, is a commercial DNA vaccine for treating canine melanoma. The vaccine is composed of DNA plasmids that encode human tyrosinase (huTyr), which is very similar to the tyrosinase expressed in melanomas. Canine tyrosinase is not attacked by the animal's immune system, but huTyr is sufficiently different to trigger a strong T-cell response and increase levels of interferon γ (an activator of monocytes and natural killer cells), which attack melanoma cells containing tyrosinase. Used as an adjuvant to surgery and radiation therapy, the huTyr vaccine has been shown to increase survival in dogs with stage II or III melanoma.

COX-2 inhibitors

Non-steroidal anti-inflammatory drugs (Fig. 19) are well-known for their anti-inflammatory, analgesic, and antipyretic action, which is related to their ability to block COX-2 (involved in prostaglandin synthesis). These drugs, however, also inhibit COX-1, which has a role in gastric mucosal protection, kidney function, and platelet aggregation regulation. Research in recent years has focused on the development of increasingly selective COX-2 molecules.

In human medicine, evidence of the role of NSAIDs in oncology emerged in epidemiological studies of gastrointestinal tumours that found these drugs to be associated with a lower incidence of epithelial tumours. Although the specific mechanism of action is still unknown, higher COX-2 expression has been observed in certain malignant tumours (Table 3). The link between COX-2 overexpression and carcinogenesis is probably related to the association between COX-2 and angiogenesis.

Table 3. COX-2 immunohistochemical expression (%) in various spontaneous tumours.

Spontaneous tumour	COX-2 expression in dogs	COX-2 expression in cats
Squamous cell carcinoma	65–100 %	Oral SCC 9–82 %
Oral melanoma	60 %	
Prostate cancer	56–86 %	
Transitional cell carcinoma	58–100 %	37–100 %
Canine mammary carcinoma	Depending on histological subtype, increased expression is associated with greater malignancy	
Feline mammary carcinoma		87–96 %
Intestinal carcinoma	65 %	
Nasal carcinoma	71–87 %	
Ovarian carcinoma	81 %	
Osteosarcoma	23–79 %	

Numerous publications in recent years have shown an association between COX-2 expression and prognosis in several tumours. Of particular note is the close relationship between this isoenzyme and malignancy and poor prognosis in breast tumours (Fig. 19).

Another study on the use of firocoxib and cisplatin in the management of TCC showed higher remission rates when cisplatin was combined with firocoxib than when it was used in isolation. Firocoxib has also been used to treat SCC in metronomic therapy and more recently to treat canine mammary tumours, among others.

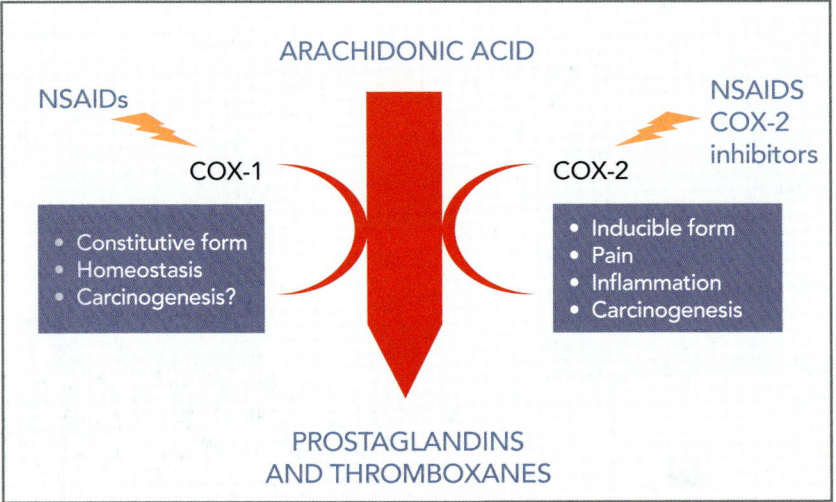

Figure 19. COX-1 and COX-2 isoenzymes and their role in inflammation.

6

Pain in veterinary oncology

Pain is one of the most important factors to consider when deciding whether or not to recommend euthanasia, particularly in certain diseases. Based on data from human medicine, 75 % of dogs and cats with cancer will experience pain and therefore the use of analgesics is an important consideration in veterinary oncology.

Evaluating pain in a patient with cancer

Most tumours will cause pain at some stage. There are four main factors responsible for this pain:
- The tumour itself (presence or growth).
- Concomitant conditions (metastases).
- Overall weakness caused by the tumour.
- Treatment.

At times, the pain can increase as the tumour grows, and not all animals display evident signs of suffering in the initial stages.

It is therefore important to evaluate and classify pain at each stage of disease and to adapt the use of analgesics accordingly.

Although pain can be classified in many ways, one very general but useful system is to differentiate between nociceptive and neuropathic pain.
- **Nociceptive pain** can additionally be classified as **somatic** (affecting the skin and musculoskeletal system and easy to locate) or **visceral** (affecting internal organs and more difficult to locate). Signs of nociceptive pain are easily recognisable by both owners and veterinary surgeons.
- **Neuropathic pain** is caused by direct injury to the nervous system and is difficult to both diagnose and treat. It addition, its signs are difficult to recognise by owners and veterinary surgeons.

Patients with cancer can experience both nociceptive and neuropathic pain and it is important thus to recognise and correctly identify the origin of the pain and to treat it accordingly (Fig. 1).

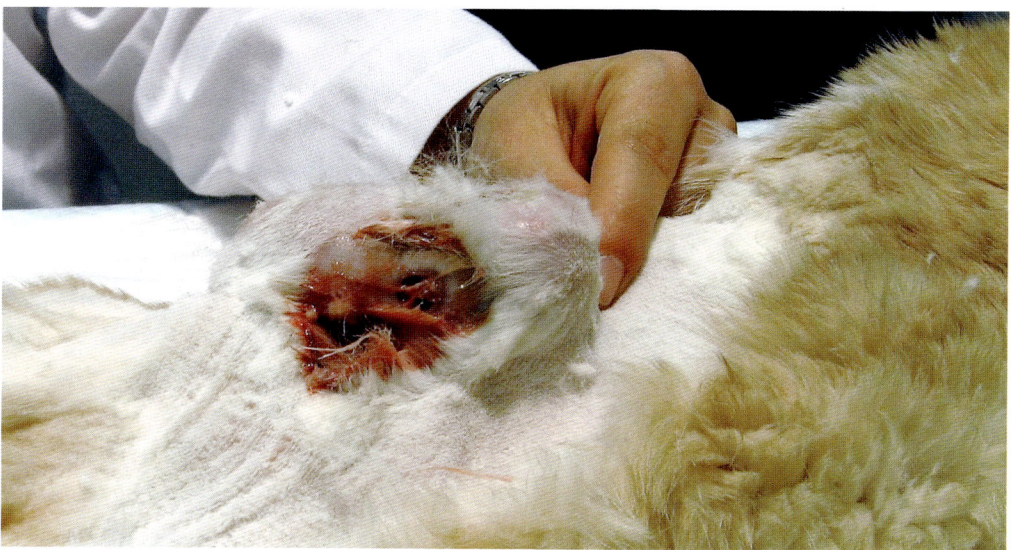

Figure 1. Ulcerated tumour associated with severe pain in a cat.

Peripheral sensitisation and central sensitisation are two important concepts for understanding pain.
- **Peripheral sensitisation.** Tissue injury by any agent triggers a local inflammatory response characterised by the release of a large number of inflammatory mediators that increasingly reduce an animal's pain threshold.
- **Central sensitisation.** Long-term exposure to a painful stimulus can result in decreased central pain sensitisation over time due to the plasticity of the central nervous system components of the pain transmission pathway.

Failure to implement early treatment can thus result in decreased pain sensitisation, making it more difficult to adequately control pain.

The presence and severity of pain must be evaluated throughout all stages of disease before deciding on any treatment. This assessment is known as a pain assessment and it can form part of a general evaluation or, like in human medicine, be done separately by a pain specialist.

Signs of pain

Different scales exist for assessing acute pain, postoperative pain, and even chronic pain. However, there are no validated scales for assessing oncological pain in animals in general.

Clinicians thus need to be familiar with the typical signs and the different analgesics and techniques available. These signs are as follows:
- **Clinical signs of pain** (highly variable in dogs and cats)
  - Posture: protection or keeping weight off painful area, abdominal defence.
  - Behaviour: aggressiveness, apathy.
  - Vocalisation: howling, purring, hissing.
  - Locomotion: lameness, difficulty running or jumping.
  - Inappropriate behaviour: self-mutilation, loss of appetite, changes in grooming habits.

- **Systemic signs of pain**
  - Cardiovascular: tachycardia, hypertension.
  - Respiratory: hypoventilation, atelectasis, hypoxaemia.
  - Haematological: hypercoagulability, increased platelet adhesion, reduced fibrinolysis.
  - Immunological: leukocytosis.
  - Gastrointestinal: ileus, gastric hypersecretion, stress ulcer.
  - Endocrine: increased catabolism, reduced anabolism.
  - Urinary: urinary retention.

Animals with cancer display signs of both chronic and acute pain. While chronic pain is much more common, it can be accompanied by acute pain. It is important to recognise both signs in order to determine whether the animal is experiencing mainly chronic pain or mainly acute pain.
- **Clinical signs of acute pain**
  - Increased heart rate.
  - Increased respiratory rate.
  - Increased blood pressure.
  - Pupil dilation.
  - Unease/distress.
  - Immobility.

- **Clinical signs of chronic pain**
  - Sleep disorders.
  - Irritability/aggressiveness.
  - Loss of appetite.
  - Constipation.
  - Reduced activity.
  - Behavioural changes.

- **Clinical signs of neuropathic pain** (acute or chronic and common in cancer patients)
  - Sudden onset of acute pain.
  - Itching or self-mutilation in a specific area.
  - Sudden hyperexcitability.
  - Electric shock–like sensations.

Pain is sometimes the most evident manifestation of certain tumours, but it is also responsible for many of the systemic changes that occur during the course of disease. It is therefore essential to carefully assess the level of pain an animal is experiencing and to contemplate this in the overall assessment of quality of life. This assessment forms an important part of the general health assessment, but it is also important for evaluating treatment effectiveness over time. Both pain and quality of life should therefore be assessed regularly throughout treatment. A quality-of-life scale can be used to assess level of pain and response to treatment (Tables 1 and 2).

Table 1. Quality-of-life scale.

Concept	Item	Score
Life activity: • 0 (very poor) • to 100 (excellent)	Mental status	0 to 100
	General activity level	0 to 100
	Appetite	0 to 100
	Defecation	0 to 100
	Urination	0 to 100
	Overall well-being	0 to 100
	Life activity score subtotal (add a+b+c+d+e+f)	0 to 100
Pain score	Amount of pain: • 0 (no pain) • to 100 (severe pain)	0 to 100
Quality of life	Life activity score subtotal – pain score × 2)	-200 to 600

Table 2. Assessing quality of life based on the results calculated according to Table 1.

Overall quality of life	Quality of life
>500	Excellent
400–500	Good
300-399	Moderate
100–299	Poor
<100	Poor (consider recommending compassionate euthanasia)

Pain treatment

Oncological pain should be treated using a multimodal analgesic protocol (combination of different classes of analgesics) and even a multidisciplinary approach (combination of conventional/pharmacological treatments and alternative treatments, such as acupuncture, rehabilitation, etc.).

According to the World Health Organization's (WHO) analgesic ladder, there are four steps for treating pain:
- Step 1: Nonsteroidal anti-inflammatory drugs (NSAIDs) with or without adjuvants.
- Step 2: weak opioids + step 1.
- Step 3: strong opioids + step 2.
- Step 4: invasive techniques + step 3.

In veterinary medicine, this ladder is tailored to the individual patient, and it is not always necessary to start at step 1, as many patients may already be in considerable pain by the time they are seen.

Why treat and when?

Nowadays, it is hard to imagine a clinical veterinary surgeon who would not consider treating an animal in pain. The problem with cancer pain, however, is that it can be masked by other signs or conditions and go unnoticed. If there are doubts as to whether or not a patient is in pain, its response to the administration of an analgesic (e.g. an NSAID) can be assessed.

The main reasons for the early treatment of pain are both ethical and clinical. Clinically, early treatment prevents central and peripheral sensitisation and may also reduce the risk of metastasis. Empirical and clinical studies in humans have shown that pain can suppress immune functions by reducing the activity of natural killer cells.

Classification of analgesics

There are three main groups of analgesics: NSAIDS, opioids, and adjuvants (Table 3). The recommended oral doses for the main drugs are shown in Table 4.

Table 3. Classification of analgesics.

NSAIDs		• **Cyclooxygenase (COX) 2 preferential NSAIDs:** meloxicam and carprofen. • **Selective COX-2 inhibitors:** firocoxib, robenacoxib, etc.
Opioids	Weak	• **Codeine.** Useful only when combined with other painkillers. • **Tramadol.** Most widely used outpatient oral analgesic in veterinary oncology. It has a dual mechanism of action (weak opioid agonist and serotonin and norepinephrine reuptake inhibitor) • **Dextromethorphan.** Minimal opioid effect, but possibly exerts an inhibitory effect on NMDA receptors.
	Strong	• **Morphine.** Morphine has been used in veterinary medicine for many years. Its long-term use, however, is not recommended as it can cause adverse effects, such as constipation and urinary retention. It has an immunosuppressive effect. • **Buprenorphine.** Lower analgesic effect than morphine. It can cause anorexia in dogs and cats in the medium term. Sublingual use of the injectable form is associated with a bioavailability of close to 100 % in cats and 40 % in dogs. The tablet form should not be used as it has an absorption of just 7 %. • **Fentanyl** (transdermal use only). Administered via patches that are replaced every 3–4 days. Highly variable absorption.
Adjuvants		• **Amantadine:** NMDA (N-methyl-D-aspartate) receptor antagonist with an antihyperalgesic effect. • **Amitriptyline:** serotonin reuptake inhibitor with an analgesic effect when administered at low doses. Administer with caution when used in combination with tramadol. • **Gabapentin:** particularly indicated for neuropathic pain. • **Pregabalin:** successor of gabapentin; has a better pharmacological profile for use in veterinary medicine. • **Metamizole:** can now be combined with NSAIDs (was originally mistaken for an NSAID). • **Paracetamol:** can be combined with tramadol, codeine, and NSAIDs. **Never** use in cats. • **Corticosteroids:** although their use is controversial, mainly because of the numerous associated adverse effects, corticosteroids are sometimes good coadjuvants for the treatment of oncological pain.

Table 4. Oral analgesics and recommended doses.

Drug	Dose (dog/cat)
Amantadine	3–5 mg/kg/24 h
Amitriptyline	0.5–2 mg/kg/24 h
Codeine	1–2 mg/kg/8 h
Buprenorphine	10–20 μg/kg/8 h (oral mucosal delivery)
Dextromethorphan	1–2 mg/kg/8 h
Gabapentin	5–20 mg/kg/8 h (dogs) 5–10 mg/kg/8 h (cats)
Pregabalin	4 mg/kg/12 h
Metamizole	25–35 mg/kg/8 h
Paracetamol	10–15 mg/kg/8–12 h (**dogs only**)
Tramadol	2–5 mg/kg/6–12 h

New analgesic techniques

Recent years have seen the emergence of new "invasive analgesic" techniques in human medicine, although these are considered to be the last step in the WHO's analgesic ladder. Considering, however, that many veterinary oncology patients may have been experiencing pain for a considerable time prior to diagnosis, these techniques represent a potentially important pain relief tool. Below is a brief description of the main techniques used.

> Some invasive analgesic techniques are gaining wide acceptance, as they can sometimes increase life expectancy by achieving sufficient pain control (e.g. epidural blocks).

Continuous parenteral administration. Intravenous or even subcutaneous administration of analgesics through easy-to-use elastomeric pumps that allow patients to lead a normal life. These pumps are typically used to administer opioids combined with an adjuvant agent, such as lidocaine or ketamine. They need to be refilled or replaced every 3–4 days.

Epidural-spinal administration. Used to administer drugs via the spine or epidural space. This technique is complex as it requires the insertion of a continuous infusion catheter in the epidural space, which, in turn, requires very careful handling by the pet owner. The main advantage of epidural-spinal administration is that it requires lower doses, reducing therefore the risk of adverse effects (Fig. 2). In the case of morphine, for example, oral administration requires a dose of 300 mg, compared with 100 mg for parenteral use, 10 mg for epidural use, and just 1 mg for intradural use.

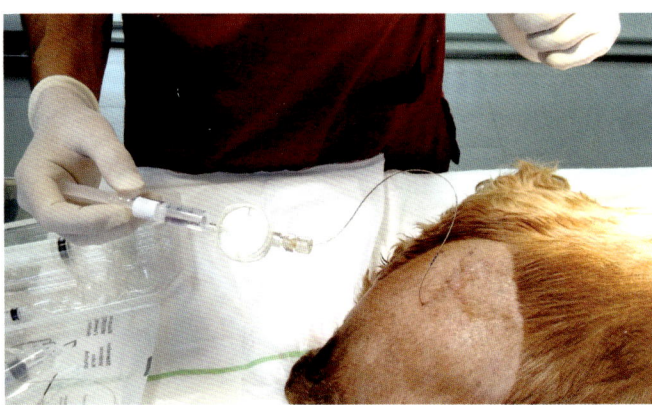

Figure 2. Insertion of an epidural catheter for pain control.

Peripheral nerve blocks. This technique is somewhat more complex but success rates can be improved with neurostimulation and ultrasound guidance. Nerve blocks, which can be complete or partial, are designed to reduce the sensation of pain in a given area. They can be administered short-term for diagnostic purposes or long-term to relieve pain (via the insertion of a catheter connected to an elastomeric pump near a specific nerve or bundle of nerves).

Analgesic ablative techniques. Most analgesic ablative techniques are irreversible and should therefore only be used when all other options fail.

They include:
- Surgical neuroablation.
- Chemical ablation with alcohol (neurolysis).
- Ablation via radiofrequency or radiation therapy.

Analgesic treatment during oncological surgery

The best pain relief solution in many cases is curative or palliative surgery. Adequate management of analgesics is essential in any surgical procedure, but it is particularly important in oncological surgery.

Correct use of analgesics during surgical anaesthesia can, to some extent, reduce the risk of postoperative metastases. Adjuvant analgesics are also important and should generally be continued for a month following an operation.

On the one hand, the reduced use of morphine and morphine derivatives is associated with higher success rates and increased life expectancy, while on the other, the use of locoregional anaesthetic techniques in human medicine has been associated with lower rates of metastasis and longer life expectancy.

Both of these strategies are currently possible in veterinary medicine and therefore pain control and relief must be one of the goals of anaesthesia in oncological surgery.

Different types of anaesthetic blocks are used depending on the location of the tumour:
- **Forelimb:** brachial plexus block, RUMM (radial, ulna, medial, and musculocutaneous nerve) block, and local injections (Fig. 3).

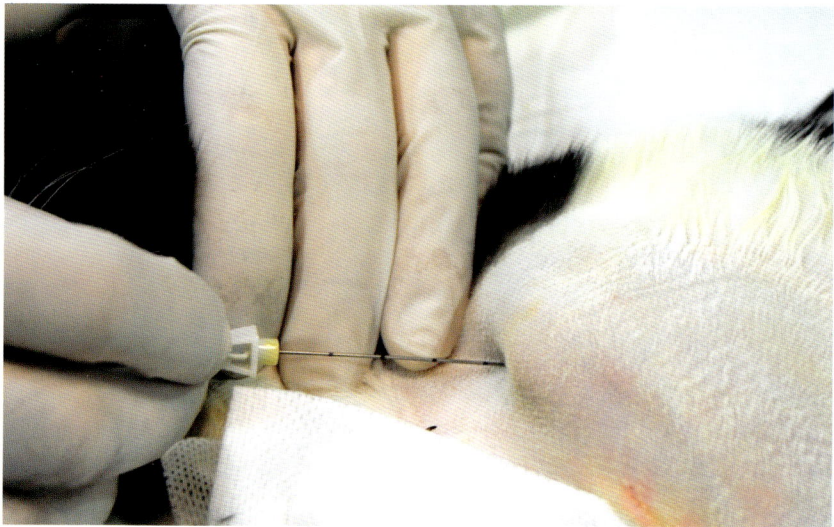

Figure 3. Brachial plexus block in a cat before amputation of forelimb.

- **Rear limb:** epidural, sciatic, and femoral nerve blocks and local injections.
- **Thorax:** epidural, paravertebral, intercostal, and interpleural blocks, and local injections (Figs. 4 and 5).

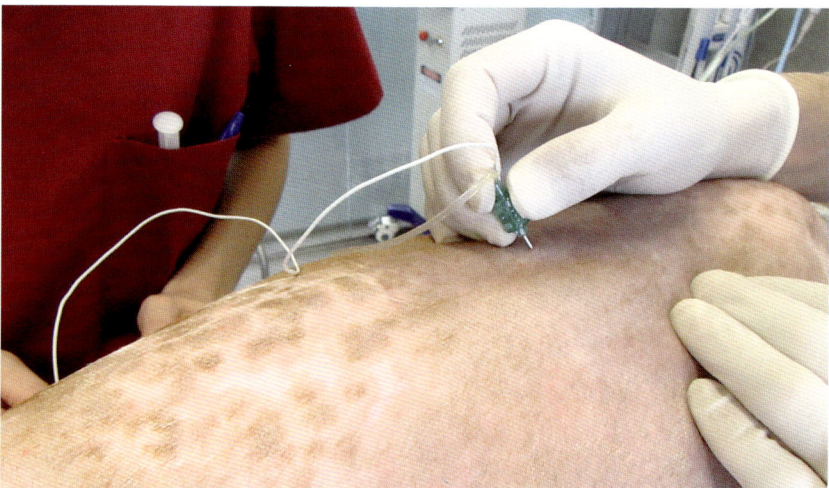

Figure 4. Paravertebral block for a thoracotomy.

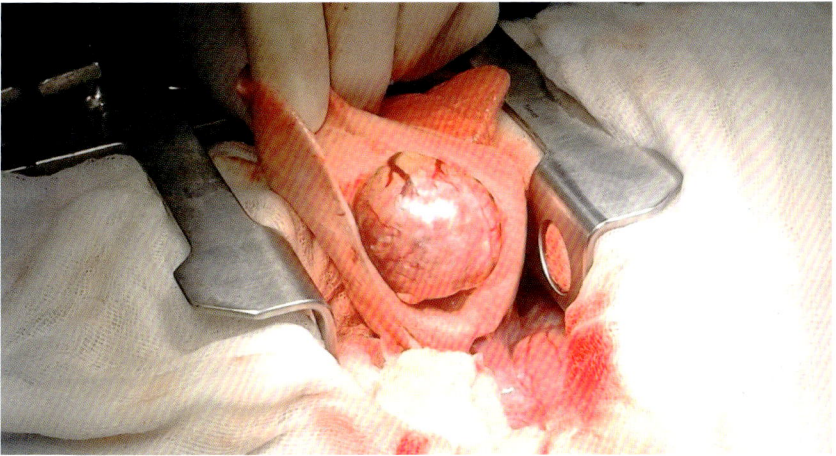

Figure 5. Excision of a primary lung tumour via lateral thoracotomy.

- **Head and face:** inferior alveolar, infraorbital, maxillary, palatine, mandibular, ophthalmic, and auriculopalpebral nerve blocks.
- **Other sites:** infiltration anaesthesia (periodic injections or continuous infusion). Catheters can be inserted in the surgical area for periodic or continuous administration of local anaesthesia following surgery.

Long-lasting anaesthetics (e.g. bupivacaine, with or without adjuvants, such as dexmedetomidine, adrenaline, and corticosteroids) are frequently recommended as they relieve pain during surgery and in the immediate postoperative period. Long-lasting continuous blocks can also be achieved by inserting a fenestrated catheter in the surgical area for the subsequent injection of anaesthetics in the outpatient clinic (Fig. 6).

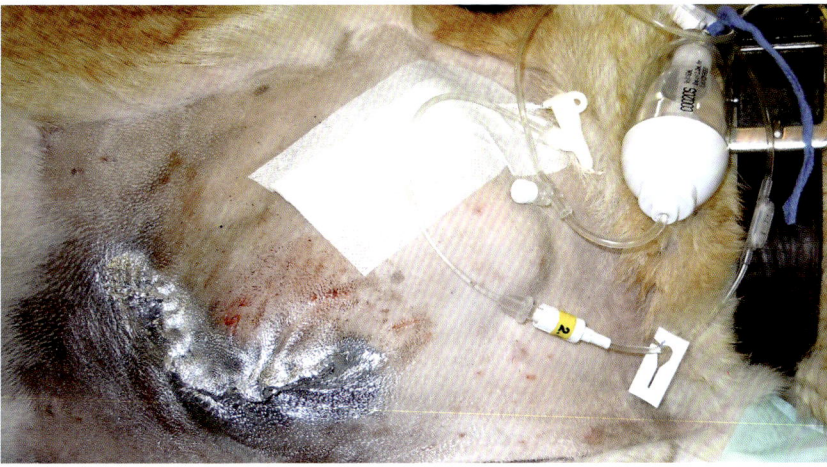

Figure 6. Insertion of an elastomeric pump for continuous nerve block with local anaesthetics after amputation of a forelimb.

7

Appendices

Appendix I. Paraneoplastic syndromes

Paraneoplastic syndromes are systemic manifestations of a tumour that occur at distant sites. While uncommon, they are very important, as they tend to indicate the presence of malignancy and are sometimes the reason for emergency consultations. They can also appear before the primary tumour is detected and may even have more serious consequences than the tumour itself. Finally, paraneoplastic syndromes can be confused with the adverse effects of chemotherapy.

Haematological disorders
Red blood cells
Anaemia
Anaemia is the most common paraneoplastic condition. There are different types:
- Anaemia of chronic disease. This is the common type. It is normocytic, normochromic and is generally mild or moderate. It tends to resolve once the tumour has been controlled.
- Myelophthisic anaemia. Nonregenerative form of anaemia caused by tumour invasion of bone marrow. It tends to be accompanied by neutropaenia and/or thrombocytopaenia and is common in myeloproliferative and lymphoproliferative disorders.
- Hyperestrogenism-related aplastic anaemia. Moderate to severe nonregenerative form of anaemia normally caused by a Sertoli cell tumour.
- Haemolytic anaemia. Form of anaemia due to haemolysis. There are two types:
  - Immune haemolytic anaemia (can occur in T-cell lymphoma [T-cell LSA]).
  - Microangiopathic anaemia (caused by endothelial lesions). Schistocytes and/or acanthocytes are often seen in the blood smear. Common in haemangiosarcoma (HSA).
- Haemorrhagic anaemia
  - Bleeding from the tumour (ulcers) or self-trauma.
  - Gastric bleeding due to a gastric ulcer. In patients with chronic bleeding, haemorrhagic anaemia will progress to normocytic normochromic/hypochromic anaemia. Common in gastrinomas and in mast cell tumour (MCT) due to the release of histamine.
  - Anaemia due to coagulation disorders, such as disseminated intravascular coagulation (HSA, inflammatory mammary carcinoma) and platelet dysfunction (hyperviscosity in tumours with considerably increased immunoglobulin expression, such as T-cell LSA and multiple myeloma [MM]).

Erythrocytosis
Uncommon. Other red blood cell disorders of note include:
- Polycythaemia vera (a direct consequence of the tumour).

- Secretion of erythropoietin or similar substances (e.g. in renal tumours).
- Chronic tissue hypoxia (lung tumours).

Other tumours that can present with erythrocytosis are LSA, liver tumours, nasal tumours, and transmissible venereal tumour.

White blood cells
Leukocytosis is common in lymphoproliferative and myeloproliferative disorders, but it is not considered a paraneoplastic syndrome.
- Neutrophilia can occur in LSA, rectal polyps, renal carcinomas, and metastatic fibrosarcoma (FSA). These alterations can cause confusion with chronic myeloid leukaemia, but they tend to disappear when the tumour is excised.
- Eosinophilia is very rare, and has been observed in mammary carcinoma, T-cell LSA, and oral FSA.

Platelets
Thrombocytopaenia is a common finding in lymphoproliferative disorders, HSA, and to a lesser extent, solid tumours. It is caused by platelet destruction or by thrombopoietin sequestration or reduced thrombopoietin production.

Metabolic, digestive, and endocrine-related disorders
- **Cancer cachexia.** Common in oncological patients. It involves weight loss and associated metabolic disorders (which precede the weight loss). Patients with cancer also experience weight loss due to reduced nutrient intake as a direct result of the tumour or tumour spread or as a result of adverse treatment effects.
- **Gastrointestinal ulcers.** Common in MCT due to histamine release triggered by increased gastric acid secretion. Also seen in gastrinomas.
- **Hypercalcaemia.** Paraneoplastic syndromes are the main cause of hypercalcaemia in veterinary medicine. The most common causes in dogs are, by order of frequency, LSA (mostly T-cell LSA), apocrine gland adenocarcinoma of the anal sac, and MM. Other tumours that can cause hypercalcaemia are bone tumours, thyroid carcinoma, squamous cell carcinoma (SCC) (particularly in cats), mammary adenocarcinomas, and parathyroid gland tumours. Hypercalcaemia is caused by bone lysis or the production of parathyroid hormone-related protein (PTHrP), which is a biologically active peptide similar to parathyroid hormone. It is an urgent, life-threatening condition that must be stabilised prior to treatment of the primary tumour.
- **Hypoglycaemia.** Caused by the release of insulin. It is common in insulinoma and can also occur in pulmonary carcinoma, LSA, oral melanoma, HSA, hepatocellular carcinoma, and smooth muscle tumours.

Cutaneous disorders

Cutaneous disorders are uncommon paraneoplastic manifestations. Of particular note:
- **Skin reddening** due to vasodilation. Described in pheochromocytomas.
- **Nodular dermatofibrosis.** Collagen nodules in the limbs. German Shepherds are genetically predisposed to this condition due to a mutation in the *Birt-Hogg-Dubé* gene. Nodular dermatofibrosis is seen in association with renal epithelial tumours (and also renal cysts) but has also been described in uterine leiomyomas.

Other

- **Fever.** The differential diagnosis in any patient with fever should include infections, immune-mediated diseases, and neoplasms.
- **Myasthenia gravis.** Occurs mainly in association with thymomas.
- **Peripheral neuropathy.** Associated with insulinoma, bronchogenic carcinoma, MM, and diverse sarcomas.
- **Glomerulonephritis and nephrotic syndrome.** Associated with MM, LSA, polycythaemia vera, and chronic lymphocytic leukaemia.
- **Hypertrophic osteopathy.** Bone proliferation in the periosteum of long bones. Mainly associated with lung tumours, but also seen in other lung diseases.
- **Hypergammaglobulinaemia.** Associated with MM and T-cell LSA.

Appendix II. Treatment protocols

In all protocols:
- Doxorubicin
  - In animals weighing <15 kg: 1 mg/kg IV.
  - Replace with methotrexate (or epirubicin) when total maximum dose is reached.
- Lomustine
  - In dogs weighing 10–15 kg: 50–60 mg/m^2 PO.
  - In dogs weighing <10 kg: 50 mg/m^2 PO.
  - In cats: 50 mg/m^2 or 10 mg/cat PO.
- Cyclophosphamide (replace with chlorambucil if haemorrhagic cystitis develops).

Canine lymphoma

Induction therapy

The induction therapy protocols for canine LSA are summarised in Table 1 (Madison Wisconsin Protocol [UW-25]) and Table 2 (COAP protocol).

Table 1. Madison Wisconsin Protocol (UW-25) for canine lymphosarcoma.

Week	Drug	Dose
1	L-Asparaginase	400 IU/kg or 10,000 IU/m^2 IM
1	Vincristine	0.5–0.7 mg/m^2 IV
1	Prednisone	2 mg/kg PO every 24 h for 7 d
2	Cyclophosphamide	200–250 mg/m^2 IV
2	Prednisone	1.5 mg/kg PO every 24 h for 7 d
3	Vincristine	0.5–0.7 mg/m^2 IV
3	Prednisone	1 mg/kg PO every 24 h for 7 d
4	Doxorubicin	30 mg/m^2 IV
6	Vincristine	0.5–0.7 mg/m^2 IV
7	Cyclophosphamide	200–250 mg/m^2 IV
8	Vincristine	0.5–0.7 mg/m^2 IV
9	Doxorubicin	30 mg/m^2 IV
11	Vincristine	0.5–0.7 mg/m^2 IV
13	Cyclophosphamide	200–250 mg/m^2 IV
15	Vincristine	0.5–0.7 mg/m^2 IV
17	Doxorubicin	30 mg/m^2 IV
19	Vincristine	0.5–0.7 mg/m^2 IV
21	Cyclophosphamide	200–250 mg/m^2 IV
23	Vincristine	0.5–0.7 mg/m^2 IV
25	Doxorubicin	30 mg/m^2 IV

If complete response is achieved, stop chemotherapy until lymphosarcoma returns and then restart protocol. If complete response is not achieved by week 25, switch to a rescue protocol.

The CHOP/MA (l-asparaginase, cyclophosphamide, doxorubicin, vincristine, and prednisone with mitoxantrone-based maintenance) protocol has the same induction phase as the UW-25 protocol.

Table 2. COAP (cyclophosphamide, vincristine, cytosine arabinoside, prednisone) induction therapy protocol for canine lymphosarcoma.

Week	Drug	Dose
1	Vincristine	0.5–0.7 mg/m^2 IV
1	Cytarabine	250–300 mg/m^2 SC
1	Cyclophosphamide	50 mg/m^2 PO every 48 h for 8 wk
1	Prednisone	40–50 mg/m^2 PO every 24 h for 7 d and then 20–25 mg/m^2 every 48 h for 8 wk
2-8	Vincristine	0.5–0.7 mg/m^2 IV every 7 d up to wk 8

If complete response is achieved, switch to LMP (chlorambucil, methotrexate, prednisone)/vincristine or LMP maintenance protocol.

Maintenance therapy
- LMP
  - Chlorambucil 20 mg/m^2 PO every 15 d.
  - Methotrexate 2.5 mg/m^2 PO twice weekly.
  - Prednisone 20 mg/m^2 PO every 48 h.
- CHOP/MA
  - Week 28: vincristine (0.6–0.7 mg/m^2 IV).
  - Week 31: cyclophosphamide (200–250 mg/m^2 IV).
  - Week 34: vincristine (0.6–0.7 mg/m^2 IV).
  - Week 37: mitoxantrone (5.0 mg/m^2 IV).
  - Repeat this sequence every 3 wk up to wk 73.

Rescue therapy
- DMAC (dexamethasone, melphalan, actinomycin, cytarabine)
  - Actinomycin D 0.75 mg/m^2 IV on day 1.
  - Cytarabine 300 mg/m^2 SC on day 1.
  - Dexamethasone 0.5–1 mg/kg SC/PO on days 1 and 8.
  - Melphalan 20 mg/m^2 PO on day 8.
  - Repeat cycle every 15 d.
  - Replace melphalan with chlorambucil (20 mg/m^2) after 4–6 cycles.
- Continuous rescue CHOP:
  - Doxorubicin 30 mg/m^2 IV on day 1.
  - Vincristine 0.7 mg/m^2 IV on days 7 and 15.
  - Cyclophosphamide 200 mg/m^2 PO on day 10.
  - Prednisone 20 mg/m^2 PO every 48 h.
  - Trimethoprim–sulfamethoxazole 15 mg/kg PO every 12 h.
  - Repeat cycle every 21 d.
- Lomustine
  - Lomustine 60–70 mg/m^2 PO every 21 d.
  - Prednisone 40–50 mg/m^2 every 24 h for 7 d and then 20–25 mg/m^2 every 48 h.
- Lomustine/vincristine
  - Lomustine 60–70 mg/m^2 VO on day 1.
  - Vincristine 0.5–0.7 mg/m^2 IV on day 10.
  - Prednisone 40–50 mg/m^2 every 24 h for 7 d and then 20–25 mg/m^2 every 48 h.
  - Repeat cycle every 21 d.
- Lomustine/vinblastine:
  - Lomustine 60–70 mg/m^2 PO day 1 (repeat every 21–28 d).
  - Vinblastine 2 mg/m^2 IV on day 14.

- Prednisone 40–50 mg/m² every 24 h for 7 d and then 20–25 mg/m² every 48 h.
- Repeat cycle every 21 d.
- MOPP (mechlorethamine, vincristine, procarbazine, prednisone)
  - Mechlorethamine 3 mg/m² IV on day 1.
  - Vincristine 0.6–0.7 mg/m² IV on days 1 and 7.
  - Procarbazine 50 mg/m² PO every 24 h on days 1–14.
  - Prednisone 20–30 mg/m² every 24 h for 14 d.
  - Repeat cycle on day 21.
- LOPP (lomustine, vincristine, procarbazine, prednisone)
  - Lomustine 50–60 mg/m² IV on day 1.
  - Vincristine 0.6 mg/m² IV on days 1 and 7.
  - Procarbazine 50 mg/m² PO every 24 h on days 1–14.
  - Prednisone 20–30 mg/m² every 24 h for 14 d.
  - Repeat cycle on day 28.
- Doxorubicin/temozolomide
  - Doxorubicin 30 mg/m² IV on day 1.
  - Temozolomide 80 mg/m² PO every 24 h for 5 d (days 1–5).
  - Prednisone 40–50 mg/m² every 24 h for 7 d and then 20–25 mg/m² every 48 h.
  - Replace with actinomycin D (0.75 mg/m² IV) or mitoxantrone (5 mg/m² IV) when the maximum dose of doxorubicin is reached.

Feline lymphoma

Induction therapy

Induction protocols for feline LSA:
- CHOP protocol (Table 3).
- COP (cyclophosphamide, vincristine, prednisone) protocol (Table 4).

Table 3. CHOP induction therapy protocol for feline lymphosarcoma.

Week	Drug	Dose
1	Vincristine	0.5 mg/m² IV
	Cyclophosphamide	200 mg/m² PO
	Prednisolone (or prednisone)	40 mg/m² PO every 24 h for 7 d and then 20–25 mg/m² every 48 h
2	Vincristine	0.5 mg/m² IV
3	Doxorubicin	1 mg/kg IV

Continued on next page ⇒

Week	Drug	Dose
5	Vincristine	0.5 mg/m² IV
5	Cyclophosphamide	200 mg/m² PO
6	Vincristine	0.5 mg/m² IV
7	Doxorubicin	1 mg/kg IV
9	Vincristine	0.5 mg/m² IV
9	Cyclophosphamide	200 mg/m² PO
11	Doxorubicin	1 mg/kg IV
13	Vincristine	0.5 mg/m² IV
13	Cyclophosphamide	200 mg/m² PO
15	Doxorubicin	1 mg/kg IV
17	Vincristine	0.5 mg/m² IV
17	Cyclophosphamide	200 mg/m² PO
19	Doxorubicin	1 mg/kg IV

If complete response is achieved, continue every 3 weeks.
Vincristine can be substituted by vinblastine 1.5mg/m² IV, separated by a week from cyclophosphamide.
Prednisolone/prednisone can be replaced by dexamethasone 1 mg/kg SC/PO every 7 d.

Table 4. COP induction therapy protocol for feline lymphosarcoma.

Week	Drug	Dose
1	Vincristine	0.5 mg/m² IV
1	Cyclophosphamide	200 mg/m² PO
1	Prednisolone (or prednisone)	40–50 mg/m² PO every 24 h for 7 d and then 20–25 mg/m² every 48 h for 6 wk.
2	Vincristine	0.5 mg/m² IV
3	Vincristine	0.5 mg/m² IV
4	Vincristine	0.5 mg/m² IV
4	Cyclophosphamide	200 mg/m² PO
5	Vincristine	0.5 mg/m² IV
6	Vincristine	0.5 mg/m² IV

Cyclophosphamide can be spaced out and introduced in the second and fifth week of the protocol.
Vincristine can be substituted by vinblastine 1.5 mg/m² IV, separated by a week from cyclophosphamide.
Prednisolone/prednisone can be replaced by dexamethasone 1 mg/kg SC/PO every 7 d.
Start a maintenance protocol if complete response is achieved.
Cytosine arabinoside (cytarabine) is added to the COAP protocol in week 1 at a dose of 200–250 mg/m² SC, divided into 4 doses every 12 hours, or in constant rate infusion for 24-48 hours.

Maintenance therapy

- Chlorambucil 20 mg/m² PO every 2 wk.
- Prednisolone (or prednisolone) 20 mg/m² PO every 48 h.
- Vincristine 0.5 mg/m² every 2 wk, alternating with chlorambucil.

Rescue therapy
- AC protocol
  - Doxorubicin 1 mg/kg IV on day 1.
  - Cyclophosphamide 100 mg/m^2 PO on days 10 and 11 after doxorubicin.
  - Prednisolone (or prednisone) 40–50 mg/m^2 every 24 h for 7 d and then 20–25 mg/m^2 every 48 h.
  - Prednisolone can be replaced by dexamethasone 1 mg/kg SC/PO every 7 d.
  - Repeat cycle every 21 d.
- Lomustine
  - Lomustine 50 mg/m^2 or 1.5–2 mg/kg PO every 3–4 weeks.
  - Prednisolone (or prednisone) 40–50 mg/m^2 every 24 h for 7 d and then 20–25 mg/m^2 every 48 h.
  - Prednisolone (or prednisone) can be replaced by dexamethasone 1 mg/kg SC/PO every 7 d.
- Mitoxantrone/chlorambucil
  - Mitoxantrone 4.5–5 mg/m^2 IV every 21–28 d.
  - Chlorambucil 20 mg/m^2 PO on day 15.
  - Prednisolone (or prednisone) 40–50 mg/m^2 every 24 h for 7 d and then 20–25 mg/m^2 every 48 h.
  - Prednisolone (or prednisone) can be replaced by dexamethasone 1 mg/kg SC/PO every 7 d.

Canine haemangiosarcoma/Soft tissue sarcoma
Initiation therapy
- VAC (vincristine, actinomycin D, cyclophosphamide)
  - Doxorubicin 30 mg/m^2 IV on day 1.
  - Vincristine 0.7 mg/m^2 IV on days 7 and 14.
  - Cyclophosphamide 200–250 mg/m^2 VO day 10.
  - Trimethoprim–sulfamethoxazole every 12 h throughout the cycle.
  - Repeat cycle on day 21.
- Modified VAC
  - Doxorubicin 30 mg/m^2 IV on day 1.
  - Cyclophosphamide 200 mg/m^2 PO on day 7.
  - Vincristine 0.6–0.7 mg/m^2 IV on day 14.
  - Repeat cycle on day 21.
- AC protocol
  - Doxorubicin 30 mg/m^2 IV on day 1.
  - Cyclophosphamide 200-300 mg/m^2 VO day 10.
  - Repeat cycle on day 21.

Maintenance therapy
- Chlorambucil 4–5 mg/m^2 PO every 24–48 h together with an NSAID at a standard dose.
- Cyclophosphamide 10–15 mg/m^2 PO every 24–48 h together with an NSAID at a standard dose.

Multiple myeloma
Induction therapy
- Melphalan/prednisone
  - Melphalan 6–8 mg/m^2 PO every 24 h for 5 d; repeat every 21 d.
  - Prednisone 40 mg/m^2 PO every 24 h for 7 d and then 20 mg/m^2 PO every 48 h.

Reinduction therapy
- Cyclophosphamide
  - Cyclophosphamide 200 mg/m^2 PO every 2 wk.
  - Prednisone 40 mg/m^2 PO every 24 h for 7 d and then 20 mg/m^2 PO every 48 h.
- VACD
  - Doxorubicin 30 mg/m^2 IV on day 1.
  - Cyclophosphamide 200 mg/m^2 IV/PO on day 8.
  - Vincristine 0.5–0.6 mg/m^2 IV on day 15.
  - Dexamethasone 0.5–1 mg/kg IV/SC/PO on days 1, 8, and 15.
- Lomustine
  - Lomustine 60–70 mg/m^2 PO every 21 d.
  - Prednisone 40 mg/m^2 PO every 24 h for 7 d and then 20 mg/m^2 PO every 48 h.
- Chlorambucil
  - Chlorambucil 20–30 mg/m^2 PO every 14 d.
  - Prednisone 40 mg/m^2 PO every 24 h for 7 d and then 20 mg/m^2 PO every 48 h.

Canine mast cell tumour
- LVP (lomustine, vinblastine, prednisone)
  - Lomustine 60–80 mg/m^2 PO on day 1.
  - Vinblastine 2–4 mg/m^2 on day 10 or 14.
  - Prednisone 40 mg/m^2 PO every 24 h for 7 d and then 20 mg/m^2 PO every 48 h.
  - Repeat cycle every 21 days for 4–6 months.
- LP (lomustine, prednisone)
  - Lomustine 60–80 mg/m^2 PO every 3–4 wk.

- Prednisone 40 mg/m^2 PO every 24 h for 7 d and then 20 mg/m^2 PO every 48 h.
- Repeat cycle every 21 days for 4–6 months.
- CVP (cyclophosphamide, vinblastine, prednisone)
  - Vinblastine 2–4 mg/m^2 IV on day 1.
  - Cyclophosphamide 200 mg/m^2 PO on day 8.
  - Prednisone 40 mg/m^2 PO every 24 h for 7 d and then 20 mg/m^2 PO every 48 h.
  - Repeat cycle every 21 days for 4–6 months.
- ITK: masitinib 12.5 mg/kg/d PO or toceranib phosphate 2.5–3.25 mg/kg PO Monday, Wednesday, and Friday, or every 48 h.

Carcinomas in dogs
- Carboplatin: 300 mg/m^2 IV every 3 wk. Administer 4–6 cycles.
- Mitoxantrone: 5 mg/m^2 IV every 3 wk together with an NSAID. Administer until tumour is under control.
- FAC (5-fluorouracil, doxorubicin, cyclophosphamide)
  - Doxorubicin 30 mg/m^2 IV on day 1.
  - 5-Fluorouracil 150 mg/m^2 IV on day 8.
  - Cyclophosphamide 200 mg/m^2 PO on day 10.
  - 5-Fluorouracil 150 mg/m^2 IV on day 15.
  - Trimethoprim–sulfamethoxazole 15 mg/kg/12 h PO.
  - Repeat cycle every 21 d.

Carcinomas and sarcomas in cats
- Carboplatin: 200–250 mg/m^2 IV every 3 wk. Administer 4–6 cycles.
- AC
  - Doxorubicin 1 mg/kg IV on day 1.
  - Cyclophosphamide 200 mg/m^2 PO on day 10.
  - Repeat cycle every 21 d.

Osteosarcoma in dogs
- Doxorubicin 30 mg/m^2 IV every 14 d. Administer 6 cycles.
- Carboplatin 300 mg/m^2 IV every 21 d. Administer 6 cycles

Appendix III. Metronomic therapy

Combined with an NSAID at a standard dose.
- Cyclophosphamide: 10–15 mg/m^2 PO every 24–48 h.
- Chlorambucil 2–4 mg/m^2 PO every 24–48 h.

Appendix IV. Survival data for nervous system tumours

This appendix shows the survival data for different types of nervous system tumours according to the treatment administered.

Tumour type	Palliative treatment (corticosteroids and symptomatic)	Chemotherapy	Surgery
INTRACRANIAL TUMOURS			
Unspecified intracranial tumours	- 56 days (10–307 days) *J Am Vet Med Assoc 1984; 184:82–86* - 1–10 weeks *J Vet Intern Med 2014; 28:1165–1185* - Supratentorial tumours: 25 weeks *J Vet Intern Med 2014; 28:1165–1185* - 69 days (n=51) (supratentorial: 178 days; infratentorial: 28 days) *JAVMA, Vol 242, No. 2, 15, 2013*		- 7 months (5–22 months) *J Vet Intern Med 2009; 23:108–115*
NEUROEPITHELIAL TUMOURS			
Astrocytoma (rostral cerebrum) in dogs	- 77 days (7–150 days) (n=7) *J Vet Intern Med 1988; 2:71–74*		
Esthesioneuroblastoma (rostral cerebrum) in dogs	- 62 days (14–150 days) (n=5) *J Vet Intern Med 1988; 2:71–74*		
Canine ependymoma (rostral cerebrum)	- 37 days (n=1) *J Vet Intern Med 1988; 2:71–74*		
Oligodendroglioma in cats	- 5 days (n=1) *J Vet Intern Med 2003; 17, 850–859*		- 1–30 days (n=2) *J Vet Intern Med 2003; 17, 850–859*
Glioblastoma multiforme in cats			- 1 day (n=1) *J Vet Intern Med 2003; 17, 850–859*
Ependymoma in cats	- 685 days (n=1) *J Vet Intern Med 2003; 17, 850–859*		- 22 months (2 operations) (n1) *JAVMA 1993; 203, 1437–1440*
TUMOURS OF THE MENINGES			
Meningiomas (rostral cerebrum) in dogs	- 75 days (1–405 days) (n=13) *J Vet Intern Med 1988; 2:71–74* - 59–81 days *JAVMA 2006; 229:394–400*	- Lomustine 13 months (n=1) *J Vet Med Sci 2006, 68:383–386*	- 7 months *JAVMA 2006; 229:394–400* - 4.5–7 months *J Vet Intern Med 2014; 28:1165–1185*
Feline meningioma	- 18 days *J Vet Intern Med 2003; 17:850–859*		- 22 months (n=17) *JAVMA 1993; 203:1437–1440* - 27 months (n=34) *J Vet Intern Med 2003; 17:850–859* - 71 % survival at 6 months, 66 % at 1 year, and 50 % at 2 years (n=42). *Veterinary Surgery 1994; 23:94–100*
SELLAR REGION TUMOURS			
Pituitary tumours	- 52.5 days (1–323 days) (n=5) *J Vet Intern Med 2003; 17:850–859*		
HEMATOPOIETIC TUMOURS			
Lymphoma in cats	- 21 days (9–270 days) (n=9) *J Vet Intern Med 2003; 17:850–859*		- 30 days (n=1) *J Vet Intern Med 2003; 17:850–859*
METASTASES/INFILTRATIVE TUMOURS			
Nasal adenocarcinoma in dogs	- 12 days (3–31 days) (n=3) *J Vet Intern Med 1988; 2:71–74*		
Canine nasal squamous cell carcinoma	- 65 days (7-182 days) (n=3) *J Vet Intern Med 1988; 2:71–74*		
TUMOURS OF THE PERIPHERAL NERVOUS SYSTEM			
Trigeminal nerve tumour	- 12 months (5–21 months) (n=7) *J Am Anim Hosp Assoc 1998; 34:19–25*		- 5–27 months (n=3) *J Am Anim Hosp Assoc 1998; 34:19–25*
SPINAL CORD TUMOURS			
Nephroblastoma	- 2 days (n=1) *JAVMA 2011; 238:618–624*		- 2 months to <3 years (n=6) *Veterinary Surgery 2011, 40:244–252* - 70.5 days *JAVMA 2011; 238:618–624*
Meningioma			- 4 to 47 months ‡ *J Vet Intern Med 2008; 22:946–953*
Intramedullary meningioma	- 1 day (0–21 days) (n=1) *J Vet Intern Med 2008, 22:946–953*		- 10 months - 29 months (n=1) *J Vet Intern Med 2008, 22:946–953*

n=number of cases   † Death due to causes other than the tumour (patient with a survival of 4 months).
‡ Some dogs included in this survival group needed a wheelchair   ¥ Dogs included in this survival group had good neurological function.

Appendices

Radiation therapy only	Stereotactic radiation therapy	Surgery + radiation therapy	Endoscopic surgery	Surgery with ultrasound aspiration
INTRACRANIAL TUMOURS				
- 305 days (n=83) *J Vet Intern Med* 1999; 13:408–412 - 519 days *J Vet Intern Med* 1993; 7:216–219 - 1–174 days *Vet Intern Med* 2005; 19: 849–854			- 42 months (n=39) *J Vet Intern Med J Vet Intern Med* 2009; 23:108–115	
		- 179 days (n=1) *J Vet Intern Med* 2003; 17, 850–859		
- 7.5 months (n=16) *JAVMA* 2006; 229:394–400 - 5–9 months *J Vet Med Sci* 2006, 68:383–386		- 18 months (4–34 months)† (n=6) *Can Vet J* 2011; 52:748–752 - 16.5 months (3–58 months) (n=13) *J Vet Intern Med* 2009; 23:108–115 - 16.5–30 months *J Vet Intern Med* 2014; 28:1165–1185	- 70 months *J Vet Intern Med* 2009; 23:108–115	- 41.8 months (n=17) *JAVMA* 2006; 229:394–400 - + Hydroxyurea 42.1 m (n=2) *JAVMA* 2006; 229:394–400
TUMOURS OF THE PERIPHERAL NERVOUS SYSTEM				
	- 29.3 months (n=3) *Vet Comp Oncol* 2015; 13:409–23 - 24.8 months (n=8) *J Vet Intern Med* 2016; 30:1112–11120			
SPINAL CORD TUMOURS				
		- 5.5 years (n=1) - 269 days (n=1) *Veterinary Surgery* 2011; 40:244–252		
		- 18–36 months (n=39), 41 months (n=1), 6 and 6.5 years (n=2) ¥ *J Vet Intern Med* 2008; 22:946–953		
		- 18, 27, 36, 41, 72, and 78 months *J Vet Intern Med* 2008; 22:946–953		

8

References

References

Álvarez FJ et al. VAC protocol for treatment of dogs with stage III hemangiosarcoma. *JAAHA* 2013 Nov/Dec.

Arenas C, Peña L, Granados Soler JL, Pérez Alenza MD. Adjunvant therapy for highly malignant canine mammary tumours: Cox-2 inhibitor versus a chemotherapy: a case control prospective study. *Vet Rec.* 2016 Jul; 30; 179 (5). doi: 10.1136/vr.103398. Epub 2016 Jul 4.

Bergman PJ. Cancer immunotherapy. *Top Companion Anim Med.* 2009 Aug; 24(3):130–136.

Bergman PJ. Small intestine neoplasia. In: Washabau R.J. and Day M.J. (eds.) *Canine and feline Gastroenterology*. Ed. Elsevier Saunders. St. Louis, 2013; 710–714.

Bernabe LF, Portela R, Nguyen S et al. Evaluation of the adverse event profile and pharmacodynamics of toceranib phosphate administered to dogs with solid tumors at doses below the maximum tolerated dose. *BMC Vet Res.* 2013 Sep 30;9:190.

Biller B. Metronomic chemotherapy in veterinary patients with cancer: rethinking the targets and strategies of chemotherapy. *Vet Clin North Am Small Anim Pract.* 2014 Sep; 44(5):817–829. doi: 10.1016/j.cvsm.2014.05.003. Review.

Biller B. Immunotherapy of cancer. In: *Withrow and MacEwen's Small Animal Clinical Oncology*, 4th ed.; 211–235.

Blackwood L et al. European consensus document onmast cell tumours in dogs and cats. *VCO*, 2012.

Boston et al. Concurrent splenic and right atrial mass at presentation in dogs with HSA: a retrospective study. *JAAHA*. 2011 Sep/Oct.

Burton JH, Venable RO, Vail DM et al. Pulse-administered toceranib phosphate plus lomustine for treatment of unresectable mast cell tumors in dogs. *J Vet Intern Med.* 2015 Jul–Aug; 29(4):1098–1104.

Camus MS et al. Cytologic Criteria for mast cell tumor grading in dogs with evaluation of clinical outcome. *Veterinary Pathology*, 2016 Nov; 53(6):1117–1123.

Carlsten KS, London CA, Haney S et al. Multicenter prospective trial of hypofractionated radiation treatment, toceranib, and prednisone for measurable canine mast cell tumors. *J Vet Intern Med.* 2012 Jan–Feb; 26(1):135–41.

Chan CM, Frimberger AE, Moore AS. Incidence of sterile hemorrhagic cystitis in tumor-bearing dogs concurrently treated with oral metronomic cyclophosphamide chemotherapy and furosemide: 55 cases (2009-2015). *J Am Vet Med Assoc.* 2016 Dec 15;249(12):1408–1414.

Chon E, McCartan L, Kubicek LN, Vail DM. Safety evaluation of combination toceranib phosphate (Palladia®) and piroxicam in tumour-bearing dogs (excluding mast cell tumours): a phase I dose-finding study. *Vet Comp Oncol.* 2012 Sep; 10(3):184–193.

Cohen M, Post GS, Wright JC. Gastrointestinal leiomyosarcoma in 14 dogs. *J Vet Intern Med.* 2003; 17(1):107–110.

Creevy KE. Airway evaluation and flexible endoscopic procedures in dogs and cats: laryngoscopy, transtracheal wash, tracheobronchoscopy, and bronchoalveolar lavage. *Vet Clin North Am Small Anim Pract.* 2009 Sep; 39(5):869–880.

Culp WTN et al. Feline visceral hemangiosarcoma. *J Vet Intern Med* 2008; 22:148–152.

Custead MR, Weng HY, Childress MO. Retrospective comparison of three doses of metronomic chlorambucil for tolerability and efficacy in dogs with spontaneous cancer. *Vet Comp Oncol.* 2016 May 2. doi: 10.1111/vco.12222. [Epub ahead of print].

Daly M, Sheppard S, Cohen N et al. Safety of masitinib mesylate in healthy cats. *J Vet Intern Med.* 2011 Mar–Apr; 25(2):297–302.

Da Silva EO et al. Malignant pilomatricoma in a dog. *J. Comp. Path.* 2012; 147:214–217.

Dear JD, Johnson LR. Lower respiratory tract endoscopy in the cat: diagnostic approach to bronchial disease. *J Feline Med Surg.* 2013 Nov; 15(11):1019–1027.

Decker B, Parker HG, Dhawan D et al. Homologous mutation to human BRAF V600E is common in naturally occurring canine bladder cancer-evidence for a relevant model system and urine-based diagnostic test. *Mol Cancer Res.* 2015 Jun; 13(6):993–1002.

Denovo RC. Diseases of the stomach. In: Tams, T.R. (ed.) *Handbook of small animal gastroenterology.* (2nd ed). Ed. W.B. Saunders Company. Philadelphia, 2003:159–194.

Dervisis NG et al. Treatment with DAV for advanced-stage hemangiosarcoma in dogs. *JAAHA.* 2011 May/Jun.

Dobromylskyj P, Flecknell PA, Lascelles BD et al. Management of postoperative and other acute pain. In: *Pain Management in Animals.* 2000. Ed. W.B. Sounders.

Domingo V, Ruano R, Martínez-Merlo EM, del Castillo N, Aceña C, Rollón E. Toceranib and cox2 inhibitor as palliative treatment or adjuvant to conservative surgery in dogs with oral melanoma. *European Society of Veterinary Oncology Annual Congress.* 2014; 22 May; Viena (Austria).

Domingo V, Ruano R, Martínez-Merlo EM, Rodríguez E, Aceña C, Arconada L. Clinical response and adverse effect assessment in cats bearing tumours treated with toceranib. *European Society of Veterinary Oncology Annual Congress.* 2013; 30 May–1 Jun; Lisboa (Portugal).

Domingo V, Ruano R, Martínez-Merlo EM, Rodríguez E, Rollón E, Aceña C Arconada L, de Andrés FJ, del Castillo N. Clinical response and adverse effect assessment in dogs bearing non-mast cell tumours treated with toceranib. *European Society of Veterinary Oncology Annual Congress.* 2013; 30 May–1 Jun; Lisboa (Portugal).

Fahey CE, Milner RJ, Kow K, Bacon NJ, Salute ME. Apoptotic effects of the tyrosine kinase inhibitor, masitinib mesylate, on canine osteosarcoma cells. *Anticancer Drugs.* 2013 Jun; 24(5):519–526.

Finotello R et al. A retrospective analysis of chemotherapy switch suggests improved outcome in surgically removed, biologically aggressive canine haemangiosarcoma. *Veterinary and Comparative Oncology.* 2016.

Finotello R et al. Comparison of doxorubicin-cyclophosphamide with doxorubicin-dacarbazine for the adjuvant treatment of canine hemangiosarcoma. *VCO.* 2015.

Flecknell P, Pearson W. *Pain management in animal.* Ed Saunders, 2000.

Gardner HL et al. Maintenance therapy with toceranib following doxorubicin-based chemotherapy for canine splenic hemangiosarcoma. *BMC Veterinary Research.* 2015; 11:131.

Ghaffari S et al. A retrospective evaluation of doxorubicin-based chemotherapy for dogs with right atrial masses and pericardial effusion. *Journal of Small Animal Practice.* 2014.

Gieger T. Alimentary lymphoma in cats and dogs. *Vet Clin North Am Small Anim Pract.* 2011 41: 419–432.

Gordon IK and Kent MS. Veterinary radiation oncology: technology, imaging, intervention and future applications. *Cancer Therapy.* 2008 6:167–176.

Hahn KA, Legendre AM, Shaw NG et al. Evaluation of 12 and 24-month survival rates after treatment with masitinib in dogs with nonresectable mast cell tumors. *Am J Vet Res.* 2010 Nov; 71(11):1354–1361.

Hall W, Clarke, KW, Trim CM. Local anesthesia. In: *Veterinary Anaesthesia.* 10th ed. Ed. W.B. Saunders. London. 2001.

Hayes A. Cancer cyclooxygenase and non steroidal antiinflammatory drugs.Can we combine all three? *JVCO.* 2007; 5(1): 1–13.

Heller DA et al. Assesment of cyclooxygenase 2 expression in canine hemangiosarcoma, histiocytic sarcoma and mast cell tumor. *Vet Pathol*. 2005; 42: 350–353.

HENRY CJ et al. Canine digital tumors: a veterinary cooperative oncology group retrospective study of 64 dogs. *J Vet Intern Med* 2005; 19:720–724.

HOHENHAUS AE. Neoplastic conditions of the esophagus. In: Steiner J.M. (ed.) *Small Animal Gastroenterology*. Ed. Schlütersche Verlagsgesellschaft mbH and Co. Hannover. 2008; 151–153.

HOHENHAUS AE. Neoplastic conditions of the stomach. In: Steiner J.M. (ed.) *Small Animal Gastroenterology*. Ed. Schlütersche Verlagsgesellschaft mbH and Co. Hannover, 2008; 176–179.

HOLTERMANN N, KIUPEL M, KESSLER M et al. Masitinib monotherapy in canine epitheliotropic lymphoma. *Vet Comp Oncol*. 2016 Aug; 14.

IMPELLIZERI JA, ESPLIN AD. Expression of cyclooxigenase 2 in canine nasal carcinomas. *The Veterinary Journal*. 2008; 176:408–10.

JOBSON JM, LASCELLES BD. *BSAVA Manual of canine and feline oncology*. 3rd ed. BSAVA. Gloucester. 2011.

JOINER KS et al. Multicentric cutaneous neuroendocrine (Merkel cell) carcinoma in a dog. *Veterinary Pathology*. 2010; 47(6):1090–1094.

JOURDIER TM, MOSTE C, BONNET MC et al. Local immunotherapy of spontaneous feline fibrosarcomas using recombinant poxviruses expressing interleukin 2 (IL-2). *Gene Ther*. 2003 Dec; 10(26):2126–2132.

KHAN KN, KNAPP DW, DENICOLA DB, HARRIS RK. Expression of cylooxigenase 2 in transitional cell carcinoma of the urinary bladder in dogs. *Am J Vet Res*. 2000; 61(5):478–481.

KIM SE et al. Epirubicin in the adjuvant treatment of splenic hemangiosarcoma in dogs: 59 cases (1997–2004). *JAVMA*. 2007 Nov 15; 231(10):1550–1557.

KIUPEL M et al. Proposal of a 2-tier histologic grading system for canine cutaneous mast cell tumors to more accurately predict biological behavior. *Veterinary Pathology*. 2011 Jan; 48(1):147–55. doi: 10.1177/0300985810386469. Epub 2010 Nov 9.

KNAPP DW, RUPLE-CZERNIAK A, RAMOS-VARA JA et al. A nonselective cyclooxygenase inhibitor enhances the activity of vinblastine in a naturally-occurring canine model of invasive urothelial carcinoma. *Bladder Cancer*. 2016 Apr 27; 2(2):241–250.

KOESTNER A, BILZER T, FATZER R et al. WHO International histological classification of tumors of the nervous system of domestic animals. *Armed Forces Institute of Pathology and American Registry of Pathology*, 1999; 17–24.

KRY KL et al. Additional local therapy with primary re-excision or radiation therapy improves survival and local control after incomplete or close surgical excision of mast cell tumors in dogs. *Veterinary Surgery*. 2014; 43:182–189.

LAMERATO-KOZICKI AR et al. Canine hemangiosarcoma originates fron hematopoietic precusosr with potential fot endothelial differentiation. *Experimental Hematology*. 2006; 34:870–878.

LAMONT LA, TRANQUILLI WJ, GRIMM KA. Physiology of pain. In: Management of pain. *Vet Clinic of North Am*. 2004 Jul; 30(4).

LARUE SM, CUSTIS JT. Advances in veterinary radiation therapy: targeting tumors and improving patient comfort. *Vet Clin North Am Small Anim Pract*. 2014 Sep; 44(5):909–923.

LARUE SM, GORDON IK. Radiation therapy. *In Withrow and MacEwen's Small Animal Clinical Oncology* (5th ed). Ed. Saunders Elsevier Inc. St. Louis. 2013; 12:180–197.

LAWRENCE JA, FORREST LJ. Intensity-modulated radiation therapy and helical tomotherapy: its origin, benefits, and potential applications in veterinary medicine. *Vet Clin North Am Small Anim Pract*. 2007 Nov; 37(6):1151–1165.

LEJEUNE A et al. Aggressive local therapy combined with systemic chemotherapy provides long-term control in grade II stage 2 canine mast cell tumour: 21 cases (1999–2012). *VCO*. 2013.

Lemke KA, Dawson SD. Local and regional anesthesia. In: Management of pain. *Vet Clinic of North Am*. 2004 Jul; 30(4).

Liao JC, Gregor P, Wolchok JD, Bergman PJ. Vaccination with human tyrosinase ADN induces antibody responses in dogs with advanced melanoma. *Cancer Immun*. 2006 Apr; 21:6–8.

Livinstong A, Chambers P. The physiology of pain. In: *Pain Management in Animals*. 2000. Ed W. B. Saunders.

Lloret A, Acena MC, Planellas M et al. Coxib, firocoxib, in canine cancer patients: preliminary results. *ECVIM*. Budapest. 2007.

London CA. Kinase dysfunction and kinase inhibitors. *Vet Dermatol*. 2013 Feb; 24(1):181–187.

London CA, Seguin B. Mast cell tumors in the dog. *Vet Clin Small Anim*. 2003; 33:473–489.

London C, Mathie T, Stingle N et al. Preliminary evidence for biologic activity of toceranib phosphate (Palladia®) in solid tumours. *Vet Comp Oncol*. 2012 Sep; 10(3):194–205.

Louis DN, Ohgaki H, Wiestler OD et al. The 2007 WHO classification of tumours of the central nervous system. *Acta Neuropathol* 2007; 114:97–109.

Lyles SE, Milner RJ, Kow K, Salute ME. In vitro effects of the tyrosine kinase inhibitor, masitinib mesylate, on canine hemangiosarcoma cell lines. *Vet Comp Oncol*. 2012 Sep; 10(3):223–235.

Manley CA, Leibman NF, Wolchok JD et al. Xenogeneic murine tyrosinase ADN vaccine for malignant melanoma of the digit of dogs. *J Vet Intern Med*. 2011 Jan–Feb; 25(1):94–99.

Marolf AJ, Bachand AM, Sharper J, Twedt DC. Comparison of endoscopy and sonography findings in dogsand cats with histologically confirmed gastric neoplasia. *J Small Anim Pract*. 2015; 56(5):339–344.

Martin PD, Argyle DJ. Advances in the management of skin cáncer. *Vet Dermatol*. 2013; 24: 173–e3.

McAbee KP et al. Feline cutaneous hemangiosarcoma: a retrospective study of 18 cases (1998-2003). *J Am Anim Hosp Assoc*. 2005; 41:110–116.

McEntee MF, Cater JM, Neilsen N. Cyclooxygenase 2 expression in spontaneous intestinal neoplasia of domestic dogs. *Vet Pathol*. 2002; 39:428–436.

Millanta F, Andreani G, Rocchigiani G, Lorenzi D, Poli A. Correlation between cyclo-oxygenase-2 and vascular endothelial growth factor expression in canine and feline squamous cell carcinomas. *J Comp Pathol*. 2016 May; 154(4):297–303. doi: 10.1016/j.jcpa.2016.02.005.

Minami T. Gastric neoplasia. *In Washabau R.J. and Day M.J. (eds.): Canine and feline Gastroenterology*. Ed. Elsevier Saunders. St. Louis. 2013: 634–637.

Miura T, Maruyama H, Sakai M. Endoscopic findings on alimentary lymphoma in 7 dogs. *J Vet Med Sci*. 2004, 66: 577–580.

Mullin CM et al. Doxorubicin chemotherapy for presumptive cardiac hemangiosarcoma in dogs. *VCO*. 2014.

Pestili de Almeida EM, Piché C, Sirois J, Doré D. Expression of cyclooxygenase 2 in naturally occurring squamous cell carcinomas in dogs. *J Histochem Cytochem*. 2001; 49:867–875.

Queen EV, Vaughan MA, Johnson LR. Bronchoscopic debulking of tracheal carcinoma in 3 cats using a wire snare. *J Vet Intern Med*. 2010; 24:990–993.

Robat C, London C, Bunting L et al. Safety evaluation of combination vinblastine and toceranib phosphate (Palladia®) in dogs: a phase I dose-finding study. *Vet Comp Oncol*. 2012 Sep; 10(3):174–183.

Scharmann W. Physiological and ethological aspects of the assessment of pain, distress and suffering. In: *Humane endpoints in animal experiments for biomedical research* (Hendriksen CFM, Morton DB, eds). London: Royal Society of Medicine Press. 1999:33–39.

Seo KW, Coh YR, Rebhun RB et al. Antitumor effects of celecoxib in COX-2 expressing and non-expressing canine melanoma cell lines. *Res Vet Sci*. 2014 Jun; 96(3):482–486. doi: 10.1016/j.rvsc.2014.03.003.

Simko E et al. A retrospective study of 44 canine apocrine sweat gland adenocarcinoma. *Can Vet J* 2003; 44:38–42.

Smith AN. Hemangiosarcoma in dogs and cats. *Vet Clin Small Anim*. 2003; 33:533–552.

Sobel DS. Upper respiratory tract endoscopy in the cat: a minimally invasive approach to diagnostics and therapeutics. *J Feline Med Surg*. 2013 Nov; 15(11):1007–1017.

Soltelo-Rivera MM et al. Prevalence of regional and distant metastasis in cats with advanced oral squamous cell carcinoma: 49 cases (2005–2011). *J Feline Med Surg*. 2014 Feb; 16(2):164–169. doi: 10.1177/1098612X13502975. Epub 2013 Sep 11.

Tedore T. Regional anaesthesia and analgesia: relationship to cancer recurrence and survival. *Br J Anaesth*. 2015 Dec; 115

Thrall DE. Biologic basis of radiation therapy. *Vet Clin North Am Small Anim Pract*. 1997 Jan; 27(1):21–35.

Terragni R, Vignoli M, van Bree HJ et al. Diagnostic imaging and endoscopic findings in dogsand cats with gastric tumors: a review. *Schweiz Arch Tierheilkd*. 2014, 156 (12):569–576.

Thurmon JC, Tranquilli WJ, Benson GJ. Local and regional anesthetic and analgesic techniques in dogs. In: *Lumb and Jones, Veterinary Anaesthesia,* 3rd ed. Ed. Lippincott Williams and Wilkins. 1996.

Van Den Steen N, Berlato D, Polton G. Rectal lymphoma in 11 dogs: a retrospective study. *J Small Anim Pract*. 2012, 53(10):586–591.

Warland J et al. The utility of staging in canine mast cell tumours. *VCO*. 2012.

Washabau RJ. Large intestine neoplasia. In: Washabau R.J. and Day M.J. (eds.) *Canine and Feline Gastroenterology.* Ed. Elsevier Saunders. St. Louis. 2013; pp. 764–768.

Wendelburg KM et al. Risk factors for perioperative death in dogs undergoing splenectomy for splenic masses: 539 cases (2001–2012).. JAVMA. 2014 Dec 15; 245(12):1382–1390. doi: 10.2460/javma.245.12.

Wendelburg KM et al. Survival time of dogs with splenic hemangiosarcoma treated by splenectomy with or without adjuvant chemotherapy: 208 cases (2001–2012). JAVMA, Aug 15; 247(4):393–403. doi: 10.2460/javma.247.4.393.

Withrow SJ, Vail DM. *Oncología clínica en pequeños animales de Withrow y MacEwen's.* Multimédica Ediciones Veterinarias. Barcelona. 2009.

Wiles V, Hohenhaus A, Lamb K et al. Retrospective evaluation of toceranib phosphate (Palladia) in cats with oral squamous cell carcinoma. *J Feline Med Surg*. 2016 Jan 11.

Wong RW et al. Erythrocyte and Biochemical Abnormalities as Diagnostic Markers in Dogs With Hemangiosarcoma Related Hemoabdomen. *Veterinary Surgery* 2015; 44:852–857.

Zandvliet M, Teske E, Chapuis T et al. Masitinib reverses doxorubicin resistance in canine lymphoid cells by inhibiting the function of P-glycoprotein. *J Vet Pharmacol Ther*. 2013 Dec; 36(6):583–587.

Websites

http://oncologiavet.blogspot.com.es/
http://www.vin.com/
http://www.histiocytosis.ucdavis.edu/